Intermittent Fasting + Dash Diet + Keto For Women over 50:

3 in 1

A practical guide with recipes and tips for losing weight, maintaining a healthy weight, and protecting health after 50.

Author: Keli Bay

Table of Contents

INTERMITTENT FASTING FOR WOMEN OVER 50

Introduction 9

Chapter 1: The Magical Diet of Intermittent Fasting at 50: Why Try It 13

Chapter 2: Benefits of Intermittent Fasting 18

Chapter 3: Meal Plan for 14 Days 28

Chapter 4: Intermittent Fasting and Supplements 33

Chapter 5: Other Tips to Follow to Make It More effective . 37

Chapter 6: The Intermittent Fasting Types 40

Chapter 7: How to Plan 46

Chapter 8: Diet in Menopause 57

Chapter 9: Myths about Intermittent Fasting 62

Chapter 10: Common Mistakes 66

Chapter 11: Intermittent Fasting and Exercise.................. 72

Chapter 12: Spirulina Algae: The Supplement that Helps You Fast 82

Chapter 13: Breakfast Recipes... 89

Chapter 14: Lunch Recipes... 110

Chapter 15: Snacks Recipes.. 130

Conclusion..149

DASH DIET FOR WOMEN OVER 50

Introduction 155

Chapter 16: Hypertension In Women: 5 Things To Know 161

Chapter 17: Symptoms Of Hypertension In Women 164

Chapter 18: How To Fight Hypertension 169

Chapter 19: Health Self Assessment 176

Chapter 20: Food Remedies That Protect The Arteries ... 182

Chapter 21: Tips To Keep Blood Pressure Under Control; Reduce The Consumption Of Salt In The Kitchen To Stay Healthy 189

Chapter 22: Menus to Rebalance Blood Pressure Values 192

Chapter 23: Anti- Hypertension Appetizers Recipes 202

Chapter 24: Anti- Hypertension First Course Recipes 230

Chapter 25: Anti- Hypertension Second Course Recipes 252

Chapter 26: Anti- Hypertension Side Dishes 284

Chapter 27: Anti- Hypertension Desserts Recipes 309

Conclusion 331

KETO FOR WOMEN OVER 50

Introduction: You Can Have A Perfect Body Even At 50 .. 339

Chapter 28: The Ketogenic Diet: Why It Is Called Ketogenic 343

Chapter 29: How Long Should It Last? 352

Chapter 30: What to Eat? 359

Chapter 31: How Ketogenic Metabolism Works 368

Chapter 32: The Side Effects Of The Ketogenic Diet 378

Chapter 33: The Solution To Your Weight Problems 386

Chapter 34: 7-Day Food Program 393

Chapter 35: Lunch Recipes from the 7-Day Meal Plan ... 400

Chapter 36: Dinner Recipes from the 7-Day Meal Plan ... 417

Chapter 37: Keto Breakfast Recipes 432

Chapter 38: Keto Lunch Recipes 449

Chapter 39: Keto Dinner Recipes 463

Chapter 40: The Summer Smoothies That Make You Healthy And Beautiful. 481

Conclusion 489

INTERMITTENT FASTING FOR WOMEN OVER 50

THE WINNING FORMULA TO LOSE WEIGHT, UNLOCK METABOLISM AND REJUVENATE. IT ONLY TAKES A FEW HOURS WITHOUT FOOD TO OBTAIN IMMEDIATE RESULTS

Author: Keli Bay

Introduction

Over the age of 50, it is increasingly difficult for a woman to lose weight and we are obsessed with those extra pounds that accumulate in areas where we do not want them to, such as hips and love handles. Intermittent fasting is an alternative to the usual diet, and can also become a way of life if you think of the countless benefits that calorie restriction brings to the body and mind.

The different types of intermittent fasting allow us to evaluate and choose the most suitable one for us, adapting it to our needs and lifestyle.

Obviously, it is necessary to maintain a balanced and healthy diet, rich in vegetables and whole grains and that provides all the macronutrients needed by the body, as well as the right amount of fat (preferably vegetable) and avoid junk food, seasoned and too salty. All in all, however, you can eat anything, even taking a few whims from time to time.

Fasting has positive implications for the health of women over 50. Science has shown that reducing calorie intake prolongs life because it acts on the metabolic function of longevity genes, reduces senile diseases, cancer, cardiovascular diseases, and neurodegenerative ones such as Alzheimer's and Parkinson's disease. In addition, especially for women over

50, it has multiple benefits on mood, fights depression, contributes to the improvement of energy, libido, and concentration. And as if that weren't enough, it gives the skin a better look.

To start this type of "diet" you must first of all be in good health and in any case, before starting, it is always better to consult your doctor. The female body is particularly sensitive to calorie restriction because the hypothalamus, a gland in the brain responsible for the production of hormones, is stimulated. These hormones risk going haywire with a drastic reduction in calories or too long a fast. The advice is therefore to start gradually, perhaps introducing some vegetable snacks during fasting hours (fennel, lettuce, endive, radicchio).

As mentioned, in women, intermittent fasting works differently than in men. Sometimes it is more difficult for women to get results. Physiological and weight benefits are still possible but sometimes require a different approach. In addition, intermittent fasting on non-consecutive days is better able to keep those annoying hormones under control. Various scientific evidence shows that in order to achieve fat loss, fasting must be tailored to sex.

Fasting, after all, represents the easiest and at the same time, powerful detoxification and regeneration therapy that we can offer to cells and the whole organism. Putting certain functions at physiological rest does not, in fact, mean that organs and tissues go into stand-by. On the contrary, thanks to the absence of a continuous metabolic commitment, they can dedicate themselves to something else, activating all those processes of self-repair, catabolism, excretion, and cell turnover that only in the absence of nutrients can take place at the highest levels.

Because health, diet, reproductivity, and nutritional needs are all altered for mature and menopausal women, their relationships with intermittent fasting can be very different from young women's. For instance, while young women ought to be careful about how intermittent fasting can affect their fertility levels, older women can practice intermittent fasting freely without these concerns. Therefore, more mature women can apply the weight-loss techniques of intermittent fasting to their lives (and waistlines) without the worry of what negative side-effects might arise in the future.

For menopausal women, however, the situation is a little bit different than it is for fully mature women. People going through menopause have to deal with daily hormone fluctuations that cause hot and cold flashes, sleeplessness, anxiety, irregular periods, and more. At the beginning of this process, intermittent fasting will not necessarily help, and it could even make your situation more stressful.

For women in this situation who are actively going through menopause, you must remember that your body is extremely sensitive to changes right now. If you do find that intermittent fasting helps and that short periods of fast are effective, you must also make sure to increase the intensity of your fast as gradually as possible so your body can adjust without creating horrible hormonal repercussions for yourself and everyone around you. For the fully mature woman, intermittent fasting will not make you as cranky, moody, irregular in the period, or otherwise because those hormones won't be affecting you at all anymore, or at least, hardly at all. Your dietary and eating schedule choices become more liberated from the effects they used to have on your hormonal health as the years go by. Therefore, if you're seeking weight loss, better energy, a physiological jolt back to health, or what have you, try out IF without concern and see what happens. For these types of women, intermittent fasting is set to provide hope through eased depression, the lessened likelihood of cancer (or its recurrence), promised weight loss, and more.

Chapter 1: The Magical Diet of Intermittent Fasting at 50: Why Try It

Being a woman is one thing. Being a woman over the age of 50 is another. With age slowly creeping in on you, your body begins to experience some changes. If you are self-aware and alert, you will notice these changes early enough. If you aren't, however, it will likely take a while.

At age 50 and over, it naturally becomes more challenging to shed weight. This is because metabolism will decrease, joints might be more prone to ache, muscle mass will decrease, and you might even experience sleep issues. In addition to these, you'll become more at risk of developing certain age-related diseases and health conditions.

Some of the changes your body might be subtle, but they are nonetheless veiled threats to a fully functional body system and definitely to the longevity we all seek.

This is why it is imperative to seek out measures, lifestyles, and diets that could help you lose fat, especially dangerous belly fat. Losing fat will drastically reduce the risks of developing health issues, such as diabetes, heart attack, and cancer.

Below are a few reasons you need to consider intermittent fasting seriously:

- **Weight Loss**

    A very high percentage of people who are currently into intermittent fasting did so because they either want to guard against piling up excess body fat or because they want to lose weight. That makes weight loss a primary reason for women over the age of 50 should consider giving intermittent fasting a try.

    Intermittent fasting generally helps boost metabolism in the body by promoting thermogenesis or production of heat. This will lead to excess body fat being burned and used to fuel the body's activities.

    Another way intermittent fasting can help solve weight is by reducing hunger. Thus, the stomach will always have the illusion of being filled.

    Weight loss becomes even more natural when the keto diet is combined with intermittent fasting. They both complement each other.

- **Muscle and Joint Health**

    Research efforts also proved that intermittent fasting could help women over 50 to improve their muscle and joint health. Some of the researchers discovered that the fasting period affects the way the body produces hormones. This will help strengthen the bones and forestall against things like arthritic symptoms and lower back pain.

- **Intermittent Fasting Can Help to Prevent Cancer**

   Women over 50 are at risk of developing some kinds of cancer. Intermittent fasting, as shown in research, can cut off some of the pathways leading to cancer. Intermittent fasting can also help slow down the rate at which an existing tumor grows in the body.

- **Intermittent Fasting and mental Health**

   Because of the changes in the body, the hormonal imbalance, and the uncertainty surrounding the state of things, it could be a mentally disturbing period for women over 50.

   A 2018 study showed that women who practiced intermittent fasting reported improvement in moods and self-esteem while anxiety and depression levels dropped.

   If you are prone to depression and anxiety disorders, intermittent fasting might just be the easiest way out. But you have to speak with your medical professional first.

- **Intermittent Fasting Helps with Sleep and Clarity**

    Hormonal changes in the body can cause one's sleeping pattern to be destabilized, especially around the post-menstrual age.

    It is soothing to discover that many older women have testified about how the intermittent fasting lifestyle has improved their sleeping patterns.

    If you're currently experiencing sleep issues, intermittent fasting is definitely an option for you.

- **Intermittent Fasting and Longevity**

    Perhaps the greatest bane of growing older is that old age opens up the body to more risk of developing diseases.

    Ultimately, intermittent fasting became so popular among women aged 50 and older because of how it evidently helps them live longer and in good health.

    Some even say it was tailor-made for older women.

- **Intermittent Fasting Boosts Productivity**

    Growing old can be quite a boring stage of life for people struggling with their health each day. It could rob them of the joy of living, experiencing life, and getting things done.

Older people are happier when they can stay fit and healthy. While it might be retirement age, there are a lot of things you might want to do with your life at that point, activities that could bring you fulfillment, if you're healthy enough to partake in them.

Intermittent fasting helps you experience a boost in productivity by helping to keep you fit and in good health.

In summary, intermittent fasting is the answer to many of the adverse effects of growing older. It keeps you in charge of your body and teaches you how to get the best out of your body system, effectively maximizing your potential to remain in good health for as long as possible.

Ensure that you pick the right fasting method. You might need to pair it with a diet, keto probably. You would also need to discuss this with your doctor/dietitian/psychologist to ascertain what is truly right for you and what is not. Women over 50 cannot afford to take certain health risks. So you have to be sure you can trust your health and wellness regime.

Chapter 2: Benefits of Intermittent Fasting

Until now, you must have realized that intermittent fasting is simply switching between fasting and eating. Eating is done in cycles or specific periods and fasting is followed after.

a. Anti-Aging Effect

Intermittent fasting has been proved to regulate hormones and aid in anti-aging effects. This will be natural since your body will have weight loss, more activity, and hormonal balance.

b. Helpful hormonal Behavior

The reason why this needs to be talked about is that many ladies develop hormonal problems after age fifty or around it. First, let me start with some general advantages. When you adapt your body to intermittent fasting, the body undergoes several hormonal changes.

i. Reduction in insulin levels happens because of intermittent fasting. This reduction of insulin leads to fast metabolism along with fat burning. The reduction in insulin is also vital since its imbalance can be a serious problem in women above fifty.

ii. For females who experience muscle pain after the age of fifty or around it, the intermittent fasting is something profoundly effective. The human growth hormone that is responsible for muscle gain is sped up by the process of intermittent fasting. It is relieving for people who have muscular pain. For females above fifty, arthritis is usually common. The intermittent fasting can help you relieve the pain by enhancing muscle growth along with bone healing.

iii. The fat-storing and hunger hormones benefit quite a lot from the intermittent fasting. The hormones responsible for blood sugar control, hunger improvement, and metabolism are affected in a positive way. Especially for females who have blood sugar problems, intermittent fasting can prove to be quite something useful. It has low insulin resistance and increased metabolism. I would recommend using intermittent fasting along with the supervision of a doctor as a medical way to solve your blood sugar problem. Since the low insulin resistance and faster metabolism is used to control the blood sugar, it is imperative that you are monitoring your glucose levels.

iv. There are other negative sides to hormonal imbalance which can lead to increased hunger.

Intermittent fasting comes to the rescue here! Some critics claim that intermittent fasting will leave you in a starved state. However, this is far from the truth. The intermittent fasting method actually improves the hunger hormones, causing your body to crave less and less in comparison to before.

v. Women have a part of the brain that is responsible for communicating between ovaries and the brain. When that part doesn't work well, the fertility problems can occur. Here, I would recommend the usage of proper intermittent fasting. If it is not done properly here, it can mess up your hormones and cause imbalance instead. However, this doesn't mean intermittent fasting doesn't give benefit in this state. The intermittent fasting if done two days a week can actually give relief. (You will need to consult a doctor about it.)

vi. The hormones that protect against the disease are naturally strengthened. This actually helps in scenarios especially for women above fifty. The immune system can be strengthened that actually helps a lot.

c. Reduction in Weight

There are many reasons why intermittent fasting helps in the reduction of weight. However, I will be discussing two situations here. The first one will be applicable to general health fitness issues. The second situation is specifically for women above fifty. It is related to weight gain after menopause hits.

Generally, many females get into intermittent fasting because they want to lose their weight. This is the first advantage of it since intermittent fasting will lead to the consumption of lesser meals than before. This will also allow a lower intake of calories. Several of the hormones that I listed above are involved in fat burning and it is facilitated a lot in intermittent fasting. The body fat is naturally broken down and it is consumed in a natural process. Fat burning is further enhanced by the metabolism. The weight loss is thus a direct effect of intermittent fasting.

However, for females around the age of fifty, there is another problem that usually occurs. Since this is a female-specific book, the information that I am about to provide is quite open.

Menopause occurs when the menstrual cycle ends. Usually, in aged females, menopause occurs when you have gone twelve months without a menstrual period.

The age of women that get affected by it is around 40s, but it is also around the 50s. It is a natural biological process. Yet, it is not an easy process. The physical symptoms are quite common. Hot flashes are the most common physical symptoms. This also may disrupt your sleep, causing the tiredness. It is really not a pretty situation especially if you are a working lady in her fifties. Even if you are a housewife, this can present problems. Your overall energy will be lowered. Apart from that, it is not uncommon for women undergoing menopause to show emotional issues. There are many treatments available for the issues arising from this natural process. One of the most effective methods for menopause treatment is intermittent fasting.

Usually, the menopause is followed by following symptoms,

i. Irregular periods
ii. Vaginal Dryness
iii. Hot flashes (can become uncomfortable particularly in summers)
iv. Chills
v. Night sweats
vi. Sleep problems
vii. Mood changes (the kid throwing tantrums may make you want to smack him)

viii. Weight gain and slowed metabolism
ix. Thinning hair and dry skin
x. Loss of breast fullness

One of the most common problems after menopause is unexpected pounds which you might have suddenly put up. Why would that happen? That happens because the metabolism during menopause becomes increasingly slow. This may lead to weight gain that may come off as unexpected during this natural biological process. This can also come with low sensitivity to insulin that will end up messing up the sugar and carbohydrates digestion. All of this leads to weight gain too. It may lead to depression for some ladies. The body is starting to act in the strangest manner, and you don't know how to control it. There are methods for easing the process. I have personally seen first-hand the benefits of chamomile tea. The weight gain aspect of menopause can cause anxiety and depression.

The intermittent fasting will definitely help you in the weight loss that you aim for. I am not going to sugar-coat it. It is a process that may require dedication, but you will end up getting its benefits.

d. Lowering Resistance of Insulin

The lowering of insulin resistance simply can lead to avoidance of type 2 diabetes. Some of the women over fifty actually have problems with blood sugar levels. Some of them have issues with diabetes and intermittent fasting helps in that. Anything that helps with insulin reduction helps in protection against sugar level imbalance. This will end up creating protection against type 2 diabetes. In some cases, scientific studies showed that intermittent fasting was particularly effective against kidney damage which is caused by a severe form of diabetes. It is thus an excellent method for type 2 diabetes prevention.

e. Reduction in Oxidative Stress

The oxidative stress is responsible for many issues in your body. It is responsible for many chronic diseases. The reason behind it is because it is responsible for introducing unstable molecules in your body. They interact with other molecules and end up damaging them too. This can lead to a huge increase in chronic disease rates. It is something that the women over fifty should be vary of.

Intermittent fasting has shown to be quite effective in this scenario. The oxidative stress is substantially reduced in the case of intermittent fasting.

Furthermore, the inflammation is also reduced by intermittent fasting that is another driver of all diseases. Thus, intermittent fasting is quite a useful technique in this scenario, especially for women.

f. Heart Health

Heart health is one of the most sensitive issues that require caretaking. When one reaches above, it is imperative that cholesterol is checked. The increase in cholesterol can very easily lead to heart diseases and in severe cases, heart attack. When one does intermittent fasting, this leads to lower calorie intake. This will, in turn, lead to lesser cholesterol. Henceforth, this leads to better heart health. Research is still being done on this aspect, but generally, intermittent fasting has been proved to improve heart health.

g. Cell Repair

Over time, our body accumulates waste proteins that serve no function. The process of intermittent fasting ends up producing a process called autophagy which initiates cell breakdown. The cell breaks down ends up removing all waste products and proteins that serve no function. This automatically cleans up the body.

This process of cleaning up gives way for new cells to be produced. The production of new cells without the need to take in any medication or supplement is a blessing at the age of fifty or beyond. Nudging the biological process this way to act in a healthy manner will end up giving you much better health than usual.

h. Enhanced mental Capability

Mental capability is something that decreases with time and age. At the age of fifty or beyond, it is imperative that the body's natural processes are enhanced. Some women use medicines or supplements to do it. However, these things usually end up producing hormonal imbalance by messing up by some of the already present hormones in the body. That would not be such a good thing. Taking pills for depression and anxiety is really not preferred for aged women.

Mental capability is one of the things that also increase with the practice of intermittent fasting. The intermittent fasting increases the levels of a brain hormone. This brain hormone becomes deficient in depression when this hormone is produced properly, the mental capacity increases.

i. Curing Cancer

Fasting has been proved to improve metabolism. Some of these effects are directly correlated to the reduction of cancer risk. Though much research has been done and still needs to be done, the fasting has somewhat a positive relation to the reduction of cancer. Intermittent fasting is no different. It may actually be possible with intermittent fasting to improve immunity and henceforth, aid cancer prevention.

j. **Prevention against Alzheimer's Disease**

There is currently no cure for Alzheimer's disease. Therefore, to prevent it is something that is quite feasible and the only possible solution. With intermittent fasting being your lifestyle, the disease can be prevented. Intermittent fasting can very easily lead to brain function enhancement. Intermittent fasting also leads to an increase in helpful hormones that reduce the chances of Alzheimer's disease. Much research needs to be done on this aspect though.

Chapter 3: Meal Plan for 14 Days

The intermittent fasting diet helps you lose weight quickly because it speeds up your metabolism. It is based on alternating full and regular meals with fasting during the hours of the day.

But what to eat in the fed stages of the various diets of intermittent fasting? Following a meal plan is highly essential if you want to lose weight. When you combine your meal plans with intermittent fasting, you will begin to see massive results. Women above 50 need to keep track of their meals as they face the reality of gaining weight easier than losing it.

Meal Plan-Week 1

Days	Breakfast	Snack	Lunch	Snack	Dinner
Monday	One large grapefruit and 3 Scrambled Eggs	25 almonds	One apple Turkey Wrap	A piece of string cheese	Spicy Chicken with Side salad, dressing with two tablespoons of olive oil or vinegar

Tuesday	One large grapefruit, ham, and Lean Eggs	25 almonds	One apple, Cheese Burrito, and Black Bean	A piece of string cheese	Bun and Veggie Burger together with a salad dressed with four tablespoons of olive oil or vinegar, and finally one serving of sweet potato fries
Wednesday	Zero-fat Greek yogurt and Berry Wafflewich	Two tablespoons of hummus and 15 snap peas	One apple and Gobbleguac Sandwich	One piece of string cheese and banana	Two cups of broccoli, One cup of brown rice, and Steamed Snapper together with Pesto
Thursday	One large grapefruit and	One Luna Bar	25 almonds and the I-	Four tablespoons of hummu	Two cups of snow peas, a

				Am-Not-Eating-Salad Salad	s and 30 baby carrots	cup of brown rice and Chicken Spinach Parmesan
Friday	zero-fat Greek yogurt					
	One banana and Loaded Vegetable Omelet	One piece of string cheese	One apple and a Turkey Wrap	Two tablespoons of hummus and ten cherry tomatoes	Two cups of broccoli, rice with Quick Lemon Chicken
Saturday	One large grapefruit and three Scrambled Eggs	25 almonds	Leftover cups of broccoli, Chicken Marengo and Penne	Zero-fat Greek yogurt and piece of string cheese	Two cups of snow peas and Thai Beef Lettuce Wraps
Sunday	One banana and Loaded Vegetable Omelet	Zero-fat Greek yogurt and piece of string cheese	One apple and the I-Am-Not-Eating-Salad Salad	One Luna Bar and teen cherry tomatoes	One cup of brown rice, 2 cups of broccoli and Tofu Stir-Fry

Plan-Week 2

Days	Breakfast	Snack	Lunch	Snack	Dinner
Monday	One large grapefruit and Scrambled Eggs	25 almonds and zero-fat Greek yogurt	Leftover one cup of brown rice and Tofu Stir-Fry	One piece of string cheese and banana	Two cups of broccoli, rice, and Quick Lemon Chicken
Tuesday	One banana and Giant Omelet Scramble	Two small boxes of raisins	One apple and Turkey Wrap	One Lärabar	Two cups of broccoli, one cup of brown rice and Grilled Cilantro-Lime Chicken
Wednesday	One large grapefruit and Loaded Vegetable Omelet	One banana and Zero fat Greek yogurt	One apple and Turkey Wrap	Two tablespoons of hummus and 15 baby carrots	One cup of brown rice, two cups of broccoli and Steamed Snapper with
Thursday	One medium	25 almonds	One apple and Mediterranean	Mini bag and Smart	Two cups of broccoli

	grapefruit, ham, and Lean Eggs	and a piece of string cheese	Hummus Wrap	Balance Light Butter Popcorn	, chicken Marengo with Penne
Friday	One large grapefruit and Don't-Get-Fat French toast	One piece of string cheese and small boxes of raisins	One apple and the I-Am-Not-Eating-Salad Salad	15 baby carrots and 2 Tbsp of hummus	Salad and Miso Salmon and Two tablespoons of olive oil dressing
Saturday	One large grapefruit and Loaded Vegetable Omelet	Mini bag of Smart Balance Light Butter Popcorn	One apple and Mediterranean Hummus Wrap	Zero-fat Greek yogurt	Two cups of broccoli, vegetables, and Whole Wheat Pasta
Sunday	One large grapefruit and Giant Omelet Scramble	One piece of string cheese	Leftover Vegetables with Whole Wheat Pasta and one apple	25 almonds	One cup of brown rice and Tofu Stir-Fry

Chapter 4: Intermittent Fasting and Supplements

Not all supplements can provide the health benefits you need. Taking the wrong supplements, especially while you are on intermittent fasting, may bring harm. The right types of health supplements can significantly boost the effects of intermittent fasting.

We will briefly discuss the problems with taking generic supplements, how to choose the right health supplements for those who are into intermittent fasting, and a comprehensive list of health supplements that you should take.

- **The Problem with Multivitamins**

    Multivitamins are very popular. Millions of people around the world are taking multivitamins, so people think that they are indispensable for fighting disease and malnutrition. This is, in fact, a misconception. In reality, not everyone can benefit from multivitamins and instead choose targeted supplements.

- **Nutritional Imbalance**

    Many multivitamins contain too much of specific nutrients such as Vitamin A or C, and not enough of the other essential nutrients such as magnesium. So there is a tendency to overdose on a few nutrients and not taking enough of the others.

Some manufacturers still include a long list of multivitamins on their labels, but the truth is, some of these vitamins are in very small amounts. Many consumers ignore the insubstantial amounts of important nutrients. How can you fit a range of nutrients in only one pill? Also, we need to consider the nutritional needs of each person. A bodybuilder will require a different set of nutrients compared to a lactating mom.

- **Low Quality of Multivitamins**

Each type of nutrient behaves differently inside the body. While folate is an important B vitamin, folic acid — the form found in generic multivitamins, may increase the risk of colon cancer according to a study published by the University of Chile.

This could be the reason why some researches such as a 2009 study published by the University of East Finland suggest a connection between multivitamins and an increase in mortality, while another research commissioned by the American Medical Association in 2009 reveals no benefit in taking multivitamins.

Furthermore, many multivitamins are manufactured with additives and fillers, which make it difficult for the body to absorb nutrients. Therefore, a minimal amount of important nutrients may reach your cells.

We are actually getting what we pay for with multivitamins. You may convince yourself and choose the generic multivitamins in the store, or you may add a bit and actually choose targeted supplements to help improve your health.

- **Supplements and Fasting**

Eating whole and natural foods are still the best source to get the important nutrients that our body needs. Remember, whole foods may behave differently from their individual components. For example, the nutrients from a piece of broccoli are more accessible compared to consuming the equal amount of nutrients from a powder or a pill.

The antioxidants sourced from natural foods are beneficial, but consuming mega doses of some synthetic antioxidants may come with risks such as the growth of tumors based on a 1993 toxicology research from the University of Hamburg.

Food synergy enables the nutrients in food to work together. Hence, food is more powerful compared to its components. This is why it is crucial to begin with a diet that is rich in nutrients, then add supplements that are based on your goals and needs.

It is important to take note that just because something is natural doesn't mean it is helpful. There is a tendency for some, especially the health buffs, to abuse even food-based vitamins and herbal supplements.

These supplements are still vulnerable to contaminants and heavy metals from manufacturing. Be sure to check the sourcing and quality testing of your supplements. It is ideal to check with a licensed professional who can recommend safe brands of supplements.

Chapter 5: Other Tips to Follow to Make It More effective

Intermittent fasting is not easy. We need support as much as possible and anything that can make your journey easier. Below are some of the tips that will make your journey smooth and effective.

- **Decide on Your Fasting Window**

    Intermittent fasting is not a strict time-based diet. This means that you can choose the number of hours to fast and when to fast either day or night. The fasting and eating window periods are not a must to be the same every day.

- **Ensure You Get Enough Sleep**

    When you get enough sleep, you become healthier, and your overall well-being is guaranteed. When we sleep, the body operates certain functions in the body that helps burn calories and improves the metabolic rate.

- **Eat Healthy Avoid Eating Anything You Want After a Fast**

    Healthy meals should be your focus. They will help you get the required nutrients like vitamins, which will give you more energy during the fasting period.

- **Drink More Water**

    One of the best decisions you can make during a fast is to drink water. It will keep your body hydrated and taking water before meals can significantly reduce appetite.

- **Start Small**

    If you have never tried it before, there is no way you start fasting and go for a whole 48 hours without a meal. For beginners, you can start by having your food at 8 pm, for example, and having nothing again until 8 am the next day. It will be easier since sleep is incorporated in your eating window.

- **Avoid Stress**

    Intermittent might be hard to do if you are stressed. This is because stress can trigger an overindulgence of food to some people. It is also easier to feed on junk when stressed to feel better. That's why when on intermittent fasting, you are advised to avoid if not control your stress levels.

- **Be Disciplined**

    Remember that fasting means the abstinence of food until a particular time. When fasting, be true to yourself and avoid eating before the stipulated time. It will ensure that you lose maximum weight and benefit health-wise from intermittent fasting.

- **Keep Off Flavored Drinks**

    Most flavored drink says that they are low in sugar, but in the real sense, they are not. Flavored drinks contain artificial sweeteners, which will affect your health negatively. They will also increase your appetite, causing you to overeat, and this will make you gain weight instead of losing.

- **Find Something to Do when Fasting**

    It is said that an idle mind is the devil's workshop. When you are on intermittent fasting and not busy, you will be thinking about food, and this will make you break your fast before the stipulated time. You can keep yourself busy by running errands, listening to music, or even taking a walk in the park.

- **Exercising**

    Exercise can be done when fasting, but it is not a must. Mild exercises can be done even at home. By exercising, you will build your muscle strength, and your body fat will burn faster.

Chapter 6: The Intermittent Fasting Types

There are various ways you could engage in intermittent fasting. These types have been proven to give the same effects that have made people start fasting, and some of these potentials benefits include the loss of weight and fat. Some have also discovered that it helps in reducing the risk of getting some diseases.

These are some of the types that are popular and have been proven to show effectiveness:

- **The 16/8 Method**

    This involves fasting for a total period of 16 hours in the 24 hours that makes a day.

    This method requires a daily fast of 14 hours for women and 16 hours for men. You'll have to limit the times you eat to a total of 8- to 10-hour eating window. With this method, you can incorporate 2 to 3 or more meals in a day.

    Martin Berkhan, the famous fitness expert, made this method popular. Some refer to it as the Leangains protocol. It is the most widely known because it is almost natural. The hours you skip meals fall under the time you are either sleeping or working. Most people who skip their breakfast and finish dinner before eight are actually doing the 16-hour protocol, but they don't know that.

Women are instructed to fast for 14 to 15 hours because most do better with this short-range, and during the fast you have to eat healthy foods during the eating window. The results you want to achieve won't be forthcoming if there's a lot of junk in your food.

You can take water and coffee during the fasting hours as well as other drinks that are noncaloric.

To fast with this method, your last meal should be by 8 p.m. while your first meal should be by 12 p.m.

- **The 5:2 Diet**

    British journalist Michael Mosley popularized this method. It has also been called the fast diet.

    This method requires that you limit the number of calories you consume to only 500 for females and 600 for males two days a week. That means you usually eat for five days and reduce the calories in your diet for two days.

    For example, you might eat every day of the week except Tuesday and Thursday where you reduce the food you consume. You limit the calories for breakfast to 250 for women and 300 for men while dinner takes the same number of calories as well.

- **Eat-Stop-Eat**

  This method requires you to do a 24-hour fast either once or twice a week, whichever one is comfortable for you.

  An example is not eating from 7 p.m. to 7 p.m. the next day. That is if you start with dinner on Monday, you don't eat from 7 p.m. Monday to 7 p.m. Tuesday. You can do this once or twice a week. If it is once, it is advisable for it to be done mid-week, like Wednesday, and if it is twice, it is good if the days are spread apart, e.g., Monday and Thursday.

  You can drink water, coffee, and other noncaloric drinks between fasting periods, but solid foods are not allowed. It is, however, not advisable to start with this method as it requires a lot of energy for long hours without food. Start with 16 hours fasting before plunging into the 24 hours fast.

- **Alternate-Day Fasting**

  Most of the health benefits that were revealed are as a result of this method. That is fasting on alternate days.

There are two variations to this method;

a) 24-hour full day fasting every other day. This requires you to eat normally for a day and then fast for the next 24 hours.

b) Eating only a few hundred calories. The alternate-day fasting can be very challenging, and this made the experts devise another plan where you only eat a reduced number of calories every other day.

An example is that when you fast on Monday, you eat normally on Tuesday, fast on Wednesday, and the continue for the rest of the week.

- **The Warrior Diet**

This method of fasting was made famous by Ori Hofmekler, another fitness expert.

This diet requires you to fast or eat a small or little chunk of food during the day while consuming a huge meal at night, a typical case of fast and feast later. You eat small amounts of fruits and vegetables during the day and fall back to a huge meal.

The meal is best eaten by 4 p.m. in the evening. No food must be eaten until the next morning when you continue with fruits and vegetables.

A feast for dinner and fast for the day.

- **Spontaneous Meal Skipping**

This is a more natural method than the 16/8 because there's no routine. You just skip meals when convenient.

This can be done in some instances, such as when you are not really hungry or are on a journey and can't find suitable food to eat. You can skip these meals.

There's no routine to this method. You can decide to skip your meal anytime, from lunch to dinner to breakfast. Once you don't follow a routine, you are using this method.

These methods, however, are not suitable for every individual, and you don't need to try everything before you know which is ideal for you.

This guide is for women over 50 years old, and this kind of people often lose energy more rapidly than typical younger youths so methods, such as the alternate-day fasting and the eat-stop-eat method, are not suitable for women over fifty because these types and processes require a lot of energy, which these women lack.

The 16/8 is not suitable for every one woman over fifty, but it's a good start if you want to take the fast to another level. There's no magic to it, and no one can tell you what's best for you. You have to discover yourself.

The spontaneous meal skipping is a great place to start, but the results won't be as fast as the other methods because of the lack of routine.

The best methods, however, are the eat-stop-eat and the 5:2. These two have routines you can follow, but you don't need to stay away from food, only consume small calories. This way, you fast with a routine, and the results will be achieved.

Whichever you decide to use, make sure you consult your doctor to see if intermittent fasting is suitable for you.

Chapter 7: How to Plan

- **Step One — Create a Monthly Calendar**

On a calendar, highlight the days on which you wish to fast, depending on the type of fast you have committed yourself to. Record a start and end time on your fasting days so you know in the days leading up to your fast day what time you plan to begin and finish.

Tick off your days; this will keep you motivated and on track!

- **Step Two — Record Your Findings**

Create a journal for your fasting journey. One or two days before the time, undertake to do your measurements. Weigh yourself first thing in the morning, after you have gone to the restroom and before breakfast. Also, do not weigh yourself wearing heavy items as they may affect the outcome of the scale.

Measure your height as this figure is related to your BMI (body mass index) result.

Record the measurements around your hips and stomach area, if you wish, you can also measure your upper thighs and arms.

Take a photo of yourself and place it into the journal too; this is not to discourage you but to keep you focused on why you began this journey.

Jot down all of these findings and update them weekly in the journal.

A journal is also the perfect way to express how you are feeling and, of course, what you are most thankful for. A journal is an important way in which to track not just the physical aspects of the diet but also the mental aspects too. Never undertake to doubt yourself; your journal should be a safe space for you to congratulate and to motivate yourself. Leave all the negative thoughts at the door!

- **Step Three — Plan Your Meals**

The easiest way to stick to any eating program is to plan your meals; 500 calorie meals tend to be simple and easy to create but there are also many other more complex recipes for those who wish to spice things up. Who knows, perhaps you stumble across a meal you wish to eat outside of your fasting days.

It is advised that you prepare your meals the day before your fast days; doing this helps you stay committed to the fast and limits food wastage.

Initially, and in the first few weeks, it is suggested that you keep your meal preparation and recipes simple, so as not to overcomplicate the whole process. This also allows you to get used to counting your calories and knowing which foods work to keep you fuller versus those that left you feeling hungrier earlier than later.

Be sure to include your meal plan in your journal and on your calendar.

- **Step Four — Reward Yourself**

On the days where you may return to normal eating, it is important to reward yourself. A small reward goes a long way in reminding yourself and your brain that what you are doing has merit and that it should be noticed.

A reward should cater to one of our primal needs; these needs include:

— Self-actualization
— Safety needs
— Social needs
— Esteem needs

Physiological needs such as food, water, air, clothing, and shelter.

Have a block of chocolate or buy yourself a new item of clothing to do anything that makes your heart happy!

- **Step Five — Curb Hunger Pains**

    Initially, you will feel more discomfort when hungry, but these feelings will pass. If you do find yourself craving something, sip on black tea or coffee to help you through your day. Coffee is known to alleviate the feelings of being hungry; if you must add sweetener, do so at your discretion. Know that some sweeteners can cause the opposite effect and make you feel hungry.

- **Step Six — Stay busy**

    Keeping busy means that the mind does not have time to dwell on your current state of affairs, especially if you find yourself reaching for a snack bar or cookie.

    It is also wise to be implementing some sort of physical activity, even on your fasting days. A 20-minute walk before ending your fasting period will do wonders to help you reach the final stages of the fasting period. It can also uplift your mood when you are feeling frustrated or tense.

- **Step Seven — Practice Mindful Eating**

    As mentioned, we are inclined to eat for all sorts of reasons; happy, sad, it does not matter. The problem is that these feelings related to food become habitual, so we aren't really hungry but because we feel good or even off, we seek to tuck into something delicious.

The art of eating mindfully is to not allow these habits to master your life. The concept is simple: teach yourself to look at something, for instance, a piece of cake and think, "Do I really need it or do I want it for other reasons?" You could decide to have a bite or two and leave the rest, but you may be less inclined to eat the whole slice (or whole cake) if you think mindfully about it.

The art of mindful eating is to revel in the food placed before you. Pay attention to colors, textures, and tastes. Savor each bite, even when eating an apple.

Your brain gradually begins to rewire itself when it comes to food and when it needs or wants something.

Practice mindful eating by:

— Pay attention to where your food comes from.
— Listen to what your body is telling you; stop eating when you are full.
— Only eat when your body signals you to do so; when your stomach growls or if you feel faint or if your energy levels are low.

- Pay attention to what is both healthy and unhealthy for us.
- Consider the environmental impact our food choices make.
- Every time you take a bite of your meal, set your cutlery down.

- **Step Eight — Practice Portion Control**

Controlling portion sizes can be difficult for most; society has also regulated us to what we think is the size of an average portion should be and we have access to supersizing meals too, which does not help those struggling in the weight department. In 1961, Americans consumed 2,880 calories per day; by 2017, they were consuming 3,600 calories, which is a 34% increase and an unhealthy one at that.

To help you navigate how to better portion your food, consider trying the following: when dishing up your food, try the following trick. Half of your plate should consist of healthy fruits and/or vegetables, one quarter should be made up of your starches such as potatoes, rice, or pasta, and the remaining quarter should be made up of lean meats or seafood.

Alternatively, try the following:

- Dish up onto a smaller plate or into a smaller bowl.
- Say no to upsizing a meal if offered.

- Buy the smaller version of the product if available or divide the servings equally into packets.
- Eat half a meal at the restaurant and take the remaining half to enjoy the following day instead.
- Go to bed early; it will stop any after-dinner eating.

- **Step Nine - Get Tech Savvy**

   Modern-day society has plenty to offer us in terms of the apps we can use to help determine the steps we take, the calories we burn, the calories found in our foods, as well as research, information, and motivation for lifestyle changes, especially diets and exercise. The list is endless. There are many apps on the market currently that can help you track your progress with regard to fasting.

The best intermittent fasting apps of currently (at the time of writing), and in no particular order are:

- Zero
- Fast Habit
- Body Fast
- Fasting
- Vora
- Ate Food Diary

Life Fasting Tracker

Make use of your mobile device to set reminders for yourself of when to eat, what to eat, and when your fast days are. It works especially well when using it to set reminders for when you should drink water, particularly for those who find it hard to keep their fluids up.

Making the Change

Understand that intermittent fasting is not a diet; it is a lifestyle, an eating plan that you are in control of, and one that is easy to perfect. Before you know it, fasting will become second nature.

When to Start?

Begin today, not tomorrow or after a particular event or gathering. Once you have picked the fast that best suits you, begin with it immediately. Never hold off until a specific day; once you begin, you will gain momentum and it will become something that is part of your day, like many other things that fill up your day. No sweat there!

Measure Your Eating

Three days before you fast, it would be wise to begin to lessen the amount of food you are eating or dishing up less. This helps your body begin to get used to the idea that it doesn't need a whole bowl of food to get what it needs nor to feel full.

Keep up Your Exercise Plan

If you have a pre-existing exercise regime, do not alter it anyway. Simply carry on the way you were before fasting. If you are new to exercising, begin with short walks now and again, extending the time you walk. For example, take a five-minute walk, and the next day, change the time to 10 minutes of walking.

Stop, Start, Stop

Fast for a period of hours, and then eat all your calories during a certain number of hours. Consider this as a training period.

Do Your Research

Read up as much as you can about intermittent fasting this way, it will put to rest any uncertainties you might have and introduce you to new ways of getting through a fasting day. Check out recipes that won't make you feel like a rabbit having to chomp on carrots all day if you are stuck with ideas of what to eat.

Have Fun

Lastly, have fun, and see what your body can do, even over 50. It is important to know that just because you are a certain age doesn't mean you are incapable of pursuing a new lifestyle change. Reward yourself when it is due, track your progress, adjust where the need is, and get your beauty sleep. This is another secret to achieving overall wellness and happiness.

Know Your BMI

Your BMI is based on the measurements of your weight and height; thus, you can easily determine your body mass index, or BMI as it is more commonly known.

In total, there are four categories that an individual can fall into based on this figure. That is underweight, healthy, overweight, and obese. The concept is simple: our BMI gives us quantifiable amounts when comparing our height with our fat, muscles, bones, and organs.

How to Calculate Your BMI

To calculate your BMI, equate your weight (lbs.) x 703 divided by your height (in).

Once you have calculated your BMI, you can compare it to the body mass index chart to determine which category you are classed into.

Class	Your BMI Score
Underweight	less than 18.5 points
Normal weight	18.5 – 24.9 points

Overweight	25 – 29.9 points
Class 1 — Obesity	30 – 34.9 points
Class 2 — Obesity	35 – 39.9 points
Class 3 — Extreme obesity	40 + points

Chapter 8: Diet in Menopause

Menopause is one of the most complicated phases in a woman's life. The time when our bodies begin to change and important natural transitions occur that are too often negatively affected, while it is important to learn how to change our eating habits and eating patterns appropriately. In fact, it often happens that a woman is not ready for this new condition and experiences it with a feeling of defeat as an inevitable sign of time travel, and this feeling of prostration turns out to be too invasive and involves many aspects of one's stomach.

It is, therefore, important to remain calm as soon as there are messages about the first signs of change in our human body, to ward off the onset of menopause for the right purpose and to minimize the negative effects of suffering, especially in the early days. Even during this difficult transition, targeted nutrition can be very beneficial.

What Happens to The Body of a Menopausal Woman?

It must be said that a balanced diet has been carried out in life and there are no major weight fluctuations, this will no doubt be a factor supports women who are going through menopause, but that it is not a sufficient condition to present with classic symptoms that are felt, which can be classified according to the period experienced. In fact, we can distinguish between the pre-menopausal phase, which lasts around 45 to 50 years, and is physiologically compatible with a drastic reduction in the production of the hormone estrogen (responsible for the menstrual cycle, which actually starts irregularly.) This period is accompanied by a series of complex and highly subjective endocrine changes. Compare effectively: headache, depression, anxiety, and sleep disorders.

When someone enters actual menopause, estrogen hormone production decreases even more dramatically, the range of the symptoms widens, leading to large amounts of the hormone, for example, to a certain class called catecholamine adrenaline. The result of these changes is a dangerous heat wave, increased sweating, and the presence of tachycardia, which can be more or less severe.

However, the changes also affect the female genital organs, with the volume of the breasts, uterus, and ovaries decreasing. The mucous membranes become less active and vaginal dryness increases. There may also be changes in bone balance, with decreased calcium intake and increased mobilization at the expense of the skeletal system. Because of this, there is a lack of continuous bone formation, and conversely, erosion begins, which is a predisposition for osteoporosis.

Although the menopause causes major changes that greatly change a woman's body and soul, metabolism is one of the worst. In fact, during menopause, the absorption and accumulation of sugars and triglycerides change and it is easy to increase some clinical values such as cholesterol and triglycerides, which lead to high blood pressure or arteriosclerosis. In addition, many women often complain of disturbing circulatory disorders and local edema, especially in the stomach. It also makes weight gain easier, even though you haven't changed your eating habits.

The Ideal Diet for Menopause

In cases where disorders related to the arrival of menopause become difficult to manage, drug or natural therapy under medical supervision may be necessary. The contribution given by a correct diet at this time can be considerable, in fact, given the profound variables that come into play, it is necessary to modify our food routine, both in order not to be surprised by all these changes and to adapt in the most natural way possible.

The problem of fat accumulation in the abdominal area is always caused by the drop in estrogen. In fact, they are also responsible for the classic hourglass shape of most women, which consists in depositing fat mainly on the hips, which begins to fail with menopause. As a result, we go from a gynoid condition to an android one, with an adipose increase localized on the belly. In addition, the metabolic rate of disposal is reduced, this means that even if you do not change your diet and eat the same quantities of food as you always have, you could experience weight gain, which will be more marked in the presence of bad habits or irregular diet. The digestion is also slower and intestinal function becomes more complicated. This further contributes to swelling as well as the occurrence of intolerance and digestive disorders which have never been disturbed before. Therefore, the beginning will be more problematic and difficult to manage during this period. The distribution of nutrients must be different: reducing the amount of low carbohydrate, which is always preferred not to be purified, helps avoid the peak of insulin and at the same time maintains stable blood sugar.

Furthermore, it will be necessary to slightly increase the quantity of both animal and vegetable proteins; choose good fats, preferring seeds and extra virgin olive oil, and severely limit saturated fatty acids (those of animal origin such as lard, lard, etc.). All this to try to increase the proportion of antioxidants taken, which will help to counteract the effect of free radicals, whose concentration begins to increase during this period. It will be necessary to prefer foods rich in phytoestrogens, which will help to control the states of stress to which the body is subjected, and which will favor, at least in part, the overall estrogenic balance.

These molecules are divided into three main groups and the foods that contain them should never be missing on our tables: isoflavones, present mainly in legumes such as soy and red clover; lignans, of which flax seeds and oily seeds in general, are particularly rich; cumestani, found in sunflower seeds, beans, and sprouts. A calcium supplementation will be necessary through cheeses such as parmesan; dairy products such as yogurt, egg yolk, some vegetables such as rocket, Brussels sprouts, broccoli, spinach, asparagus; legumes; dried fruit such as nuts, almonds or dried grapes.

Excellent additional habits that will help to regain well-being may be: limiting sweets to sporadic occasions, thus drastically reducing sugars (for example by giving up sugar in coffee and getting used to drinking it bitterly); learn how to dose alcohol a lot (avoiding spirits, liqueurs, and aperitif drinks) and choose only one glass of good wine when you are in company, this because it tends to increase visceral fat which is precisely what is going to settle at the level abdominal. Clearly, even by eating lots of fruit, it is difficult to reach a high carbohydrate quota as in a traditional diet. However, a dietary plan to follow can be useful to have a more precise indication of how to distribute the foods. Obviously, one's diet must be structured in a personal way, based on specific metabolic needs and one's lifestyle.

Chapter 9: Myths about Intermittent Fasting

- **Myth 1: Breakfast Boosts Metabolism**

    This myth is so tenacious that many people, businesses, and institutions claim that breakfast is the most important meal of the day.

    For example, the site of the National Nutrition Health Program strongly discourages doing without it and many manufacturers are selling their products "to start the day off on the right foot."

    One can imagine that the manufacturers of breakfast cereals, margarine, or spreads will not be frankly delighted if people start to skip breakfast. Rather, they have an interest in what we eat as often as possible.

    By dint of hearing something, you end up believing it and you don't think about looking for evidence. But as I am stubborn, I have investigated whether the claims about breakfast are true.

    In conclusion, skipping breakfast does not slow down the metabolism. It will not make you gain weight.

- **Myth 2: Eat 5 or 6 Meals a Day**

  According to this myth, it is necessary to eat 5 or 6 meals per day to make work the metabolism in a continuous way. This involves eating three main meals and two snacks.

  Eating every few hours is believed to prevent the metabolism from slowing down. Many dietitians thus advise eating frequently, in small portions.

  There is no scientific evidence that eating 5-6 meals a day increases or maintains the speed of metabolism. In fact, the frequency of meals has no effect on metabolism.

  We burn as many calories as we eat 2 or 3 times a day or we eat 5 or 6 times a day.

  The only argument in favor of frequent small food intakes could be that they prevent you from being hungry (to which you can object that you are never really full because you only eat small portions.)

  What is proven, however, is that eating often in small portions reduces insulin sensitivity, which promotes the development of abdominal fat

- **Myth 3: Eat Often to Avoid Losing Muscle Mass**

You may have noticed that some bodybuilders take their Tupperware with chicken breast and vegetables everywhere.

These bodybuilders want to be able to eat their protein every few hours because they fear losing muscle mass.

If you are not in the bodybuilding world, you certainly have less pressure in relation to your muscle mass. Having said that, muscle mass is important for everyone. Indeed, the amount of muscle mass you have determines your resting metabolism.

If you lose muscle mass, your resting metabolism will slow down and you will gain weight faster. Many people (not just bodybuilders) are afraid of losing muscle.

The fear of losing muscle mass is understandable. However, the fear of losing your muscles if you don't eat for a few hours has no basis.

The body stores fat for use as an energy source after digestion is complete.

It is illogical to think that if you do not eat, your body will draw on muscle mass rather than fat. This is not how the body works.

For bodybuilders, intermittent fasting has only great benefits. This is explained by the production of growth hormone. Click here to learn more about fasting and strength training.

- **Myth 4: When We Fast, the Body Goes into Economy Mode**

Prehistoric men regularly went through periods during which fasting was a necessity. For example, when you came home empty-handed from the hunt and there was nothing edible in the area.

From the point of view of evolution, our body is provided with an "energy-saving mode." This mode allows the body to slow down metabolism.

Chapter 10: Common Mistakes

Now that you know all about the process of intermittent fasting and how it should be done, you should also have the knowledge of the common mistakes that people make while doing the fast. These mistakes can actually prevent you from realizing the benefits and make the entire fast nothing, but a complete waste. So, once you know what they are, make sure that you do not make the same mistakes yourself. If you do not want to make mistakes, the first and foremost thing that you need to do is be aware of everything that you are doing and also know why you are doing them. This will ensure that even if you are sometimes off the path, you can easily push yourself back on track. Also, stop beating yourself up for a cheat day or any mistake that you made. Just move on by accepting that it happened, and it cannot be undone. If you waste your energy in self-loathing, you will not be able to make plans so that the same mistake does not happen twice.

Fasting Too Long Even at the Beginning

You must have heard me saying this plenty of times already; you need to take it slow. Do not rush the process. If you haven't tried intermittent fasting ever in your life, then you should start with a 48-hour fast or even a 24-hour fast for that matter. Yes, you will have to eventually lengthen the fasting window but that does not mean you have to do it now and at once. What you have to do is increase the fasting period but do it in small increments. In case you do not follow what, I said, it will be you who will be facing certain consequences and they are bound to happen.

One of the first consequences that people have to face when they fast for longer periods too quickly is that they become grumpy. They behave badly with coworkers and loved ones. And the worst part is that you might shove it away, saying that it's just your way of coping with fasting, but it is not. Also, due to your cranky mood, some people might even give you negative feedback and in most cases, that is when people give up the fast and throw every effort down the gutter all at once. Tossing the whole idea out of the window because of such a situation is not worth it and it would not have come to it only if you had increased your fasting period gradually.

The second consequence is that when people do longer fast, in the beginning, they cannot continue it after the first couple of days mainly because it becomes too unbearable for them, and they feel tremendously hungry all the time. The process of intermittent fasting should not make you feel jarred or stressed. Instead, it should be gradual and gentle. If you truly want to continue intermittent fasting for a long stretch of time, you have to learn to make it well incorporated into your routine and for that, you need to take it slow. When you start the longer fasts right from the beginning, you are simply walking on the path of disappointment and most people give up too quickly in such cases.

Not Eating the Right Foods

This is probably the biggest mistake that I see people have been making. If you have been trying to incorporate the process of intermittent fasting into your day-to-day life, then you also have to ensure that you are eating the right foods; otherwise, it won't work the way you want it to. For starters, as you might know, fasting means that you have to learn how to get your appetite under control. And this means that you cannot simply grab that packet of chips or that bar of crunchy granola whenever you feel like. There is a time for everything, and time is highly essential. But equally essential is what you are eating in your eating window.

If you make the wrong choices, then you are definitely going to have a hard time controlling your appetite. When you are relying on foods that are rich in carbohydrates, you will be deliberately making the entire process difficult for yourself your appetite along with your levels of blood glucose are in a state of continuous fluctuation. When you are on a diet that is low in carbs, you will have more fats and proteins. This will increase your levels of satiety. In simpler words, you will remain full for a longer period of time. Moreover, this will give your body flexibility in metabolism so that you can tap into your fat reserves whenever your body is fasting and does not have enough glucose as fuel.

Also, some people use intermittent fasting as an excuse to eat whatever they want when they are in the eating window. That is not right and won't bring you any good results. You have to remember that this is not a magic pill, and nothing will happen on its own if you do not put enough effort. It is true that intermittent fasting allows you to take your health into your own hands and maintain proper metabolism but for that, your diet needs to be healthy too. You have to cut down on sugar and processed foods. You need to incorporate more and more whole foods that are rich in nutrients and low in carbs.

Consuming Too Many Calories

It is important to eat the right foods so that you can get the nutrients that you need. But you should not overdo it in the eating phase. When people fast, they have this idea that they have to replenish themselves by eating an equally heavy meal in the eating window. Never try to compensate for the time you were not eating. Sometimes people end up overeating to such an extent that they not only regret their actions but also feel bloated.

Also, in case you have overeaten, don't be too harsh on yourself because it will only make matters worse. Accept the fact because you simply cannot undo it in any way. What you have to do from now on is that you have to prepare and plan your meals and keep healthy options in every meal. This will ensure that when the eating window starts, you don't have to think about what you want to eat. A very important part of the process of intermittent fasting is to figure out a balance in your routine where you can prepare healthy foods and not depend on processed foods.

Not Staying Consistent

This is probably true for everything on earth that if you are not consistent with it, it will not bring you results. The same goes for intermittent fasting. But what is worse is that if you are not consistent, then you will be stuck in a cycle where you make poor eating choices and you will be so disappointed with everything that you will not feel like doing anything about it. That is exactly something you need to avoid and for this, you have to be consistent. The best way to ensure this is to follow a fasting regime that you can maintain for the long term. You need to understand that if you truly want to reap the benefits of intermittent fasting, then it also means that you have to do it for a long period of time without giving up on it.

In case you already feel like that you will not be able to stay consistent throughout the procedure, then you need to sit down and figure out why. You need to find the reason behind it and then deal with it. Is it because you do not like the method that you have selected? If it is so, then try some other method. Or, is it because your fasting and feeding window is wrong and you are having a hard time adjusting to it? In that case, you need to adjust the timings in a different manner. Whatever it is, just don't give up before figuring out the why.

Doing Too Many Things at the Same Time

This is also one of the reasons why people give up on intermittent fasting, especially beginners. There is a saying that you should not bite off more than you can chew, and this is exactly what I am talking about here. If you are trying out intermittent fasting for the first time and you are also trying to maintain a daily gym schedule (which you don't usually do) and on top that, you are also trying to cook your own meals (when you are habituated to take-outs), then it is very easy to feel stressed.

So, maybe you can start by training only three times a week and then you can take the help of your family members in cooking your meals. If you do not have anyone living with you, then you can skip the gym for now and maybe go for a run in the neighborhood in the initial days. Once you are okay with this routine, then you can incorporate the gym.

Now that you know the common mistakes, I hope this will help you to avoid it.

Chapter 11: Intermittent Fasting and Exercise

Many people will ask if it is safe to combine fasting with exercise. I am here to say it is. Yet, some factors need to be considered before combining the two. First, the type of fasting regimen should be considered alongside the physical, mental, and psychological health of the individual. Women with existing medical conditions should not combine fasting with exercises before being advised by a medical expert. So, while it is safe to practice intermittent fasting and include exercise if you are an already active person, doing so is not suitable for everyone.

First of all, your metabolism can be negatively impacted if you exercise and fast for long periods. For example, if you exercise daily while fasting for more than a month, your metabolic rate can begin to slow down.

Combining the two can trigger a higher rate of breaking down glycogen and body fat. This means that you burn fat at an accelerated rate. Also, when you combine these two, your growth hormones are boosted. This results in improved bone density. Your muscles are also positively impacted when you exercise. Your muscles will become more resilient to stress and age slower. This is also a quick way to trigger autophagy keeping brain cells and tissues strong, making you feel, and look younger.

Exercise Is Even Better After 50

Cardiovascular exercise is best for the heart and lungs. It improves oxygen delivery to specific parts of your body, reduces stress, improves sleep, burns fat, and improves sex drive. Some of the more common cardio exercises are running, brisk walking, and swimming. In the gym, machines such as the elliptical, treadmill, and Stairmaster are used to help with cardio. Some people are satisfied and feel like they've done enough after 20 minutes on the treadmill, but if you want to continue to be strong and independent as you grow older, you need to consider adding strength training to your workout. After 50, strength training for a woman is no longer about six-pack abs, building biceps, or vanity muscles. Instead, it has switched to maintaining a body that is healthy, strong, and is less prone to injury and illness.

Women over 50 who engage in strength training for 20 to 30 minutes a day can reap the following benefits:

1. **Reduced body fat:** Accumulating excess body fat is not healthy for any woman at any age. To prevent many of the diseases associated with aging, it is

important to maintain healthy body weight by burning excess fat.
2. **Build bone density:** With stronger bones, accidental falls are less likely to result in broken limbs or a visit to the emergency room.
3. **Build muscle mass:** Although you are not likely to be the next champion bodybuilder, strength training will make you an overall stronger woman who will carry herself with ease, push your lawnmower, lift your groceries, and perform all other tasks that require you to exert some strength.
4. **Significant less risk of chronic diseases:** In addition to keeping chronic diseases away, strength training can also reduce symptoms of some diseases you may have, such as back pain, obesity, arthritis, osteoporosis, and diabetes. Of course, the type of exercises you do if you have any chronic disease should be recommended by your doctor.
5. **Boosts mental health:** A loss of self-confidence and depression are some psychological issues that come along with aging. Women who keep themselves fit with exercises tend to be generally more self-assured and are less likely to develop depression.

Strength Training Exercises for Women Over 50

These ten strength training exercises you can do right in the comfort of your home. All you need is a mat, a chair, and some hand weights of about 3 – 8 pounds. As you get stronger, you can increase the weight. Take a minute to rest before switching between each routine. Ensure that you move slowly through the exercises, breathe properly, and focus on maintaining the right form. If you start to feel lightheaded or dizzy during your routines, especially if you are performing the exercise during your fasting window, discontinue immediately.

Squat to Chair

This exercise is great for improving your bone health. A lot of age-related bone fractures and falls in women involve the pelvis, so this exercise will target and strengthen your pelvic bone and the surrounding muscles.

To perform this:

1. Stand fully upright in front of a chair as if you are ready to sit and spread your feet shoulder-width apart.
2. Extend your arms in front of you and keep them that way all through the movement.

3. Bend your knees and slowly lower your hips as if you want to sit on the chair, but don't sit. When your butt touches the chair slightly, press into your heels to get back your initial standing position, repeat that for about 10 to 15 times.

Forearm Plank

This exercise targets your core and shoulders.

Here's how to do it:

1. Get into a push-up position, but with your arms bent at the elbows such that your forearm is supporting your weight.
2. Keep your body off the mat or floor and keep your back straight at all times. Don't raise or drop your hips. This will engage your core. Hold the position for 30 seconds and then drop to your knees. Repeat ten times.

Modified Push-ups

This routine targets your arms, shoulders, and core.

How's how to do it:

1. Kneel on your mat. Place your hands on the mat below your shoulders and let your knees be behind your hips so that your back is stretched at an angle.

2. Tuck your toes under and tighten your abdominal muscles. Gradually bend your elbows as you lower your chest toward the floor.
3. Push back on your arms to press your chest back to your previous position. Repeat for as many times as is comfortable.

Bird Dog

When done correctly, this exercise can strengthen the muscles of your posterior chain as it targets your back and core. It may seem easy at first but can be a bit tricky.

To do this correctly:

1. Go on all fours on your mat.
2. Tighten your abdominal muscles and shift your weight to your right knee and left hand. Slowly extend your right hand in front of you and your left leg behind you. Ensure that both your hands and legs are extended as far as possible and stay in that position for about 5 seconds. Return to your starting position. This is one repetition. Switch to your left knee and right hand and repeat the movement. Alternate between both sides for 20 repetitions.

Shoulder Overhead Press

This targets your biceps, shoulders, and back.

To perform this move:

1. With dumbbells in both hands, stand and spread your feet shoulder-width apart.
2. Bring the dumbbells up to the sides of your head and tighten your abdominal muscles.
3. Slowly press the dumbbells up until your arms are straight above your head. Slowly return to the first position. Repeat 10 times. You can also do this exercise while sitting.

Chest Fly

This targets your chest, back, core, and glutes.

To do this:

1. Lie with your back flat on your mat, your knees at an angle close to 90 degrees, and your feet firmly planted on the floor or mat.
2. Hold dumbbells in both hands over your chest. Keep your palms facing each other and gently open your hands away from your chest. Let your upper arms touch the floor without releasing the tension in them.

3. Contract your chest muscles and slowly return the dumbbells to the initial position. Repeat for about ten times.

Standing Calf Raise

This exercise improves the mobility of your lower legs and feet and also improves your stability.

Here's how to perform it.

- Hold a dumbbell in your left hand and place your right hand on something sturdy to give you balance.
- When you are sure of your balance, lift your left foot off the floor with the dumbbell hanging at your side. Stand erect and move your weight such that you are almost standing on your toes.
- Slowly return to the starting position. Do this 15 times before switching to the other leg and doing the same thing all over again.

Single-Leg Hamstring Bridge

This move targets your glutes, quads, and hamstrings.

To do this:

1. Lie flat on your back. Place your feet flat on the floor or mat and spread your bent knees apart.

2. Place your arms flat by your side and lift one leg straight.
3. Contract your glutes as you lift your hips into a bridge position with your arms still in position. Hold for about 2 to 3 seconds and drop your hips to the mat. Repeat about ten times before switching your leg. Do the same again.

Bent-Over Row

This targets your back muscles and spine.

To do this:

1. Hold dumbbells in both hands and stand behind a sturdy object (for example, a chair). Bend forward and rest your head on the chosen object. Relax your neck and slightly bend your knees. With both palms facing each other pull, the dumbbells to touch your ribs. Hold the position for about 2 to 5 seconds and slowly return to the starting position. Repeat 10 to 15 times.

Basic Ab

A distended belly is a common occurrence in older women. This exercise can strengthen and tighten the abdominal muscles bringing them inward toward your spine.

To perform this:

1. Lie on your back with your feet firmly planted on the floor and your knees bent. Relax your upper body and rest your hands on your thighs.
2. As you exhale, lift yourself upward off the mat or floor. Stop the upward movement when your hands are resting on your knees. Hold the position for about 2 to 5 seconds and then slowly return to the starting position. Repeat for about 20 to 30 times.

Chapter 12: Spirulina Algae: The Supplement that Helps You Fast

Spirulina (pronounced spear-uh-lee-nun) is an edible type of cyanobacteria, single-celled, blue-green microalgae that are found naturally in both salt and freshwaters. These spiral-shaped microalgae are cultivated and harvested throughout the world as both a supplement and whole food. Because it has a soft cell wall made of protein and complex sugars, it can be digested efficiently. It is widely considered a green superfood with positive health benefits because of its richness in:

- Protein (dried spirulina contains between 50% to 70% protein)
- Minerals (especially Iron and Manganese)
- Vitamins (especially Vitamins B1, and B2)
- Carotenoids
- Antioxidants

Spirulina is used internationally in nutrition drinks, pasta, crackers, noodles, nutrition bars, broths, cakes, pet foods, and cereal. It is also used as a component in food coloring, cosmetics, skin creams, shampoos, personal care products, and more. Spirulina can be purchased at most specialty nutrition stores, some supermarket chains, as well as online. It is typically sold in powder or tablet form.

As food, eating spirulina is nothing new. Historians indicate that spirulina as part of the diet of the Kamen Empire of Chad in the ninth century (AD/CE). In 1519, Hernando Cortez and his Spanish Conquistadors observed that spirulina was eaten by Aztecs around Lake Texcoco, which is modern-day Mexico City. Today, more than one thousand metric tons of spirulina is harvested worldwide in natural lakes, commercial farms, village farms, and family microforms.

Spirulina farming is much more environmentally friendly compared to conventional food production. Most conventional foods are generated using chemicals, including pesticides, antibiotics, preservatives, additives, and fungicides. Not only have these chemicals been shown to have negative impacts on health, but they also cause damage to our water supply and the overall natural environment. Harvesting spirulina offers more nutrition per acre and doesn't incur environmental costs associated with toxic cleanup, water treatment, or subsidies that other food industries require.

The growing popularity of spirulina as a green superfood has taken off over the past forty years. Scientific research conducted in recent decades supports the many health benefits of spirulina, adding to its growing use as a food or supplement. Research is ongoing, and in some cases, has not been tested on human subjects. Additionally, the U.S. FDA has not approved spirulina as a medicine or treatment for diseases (although it is an approved supplement and food). However, the health benefits that research has uncovered so far have been very positive, showing some transformative results.

- **Cancer Fighter**

    Spirulina is high in beta-carotene, a type of phytochemical, that is believed to help protect the body against free radicals that can come from various forms of pollution, including cigarette smoke and herbicides. Spirulina's effects on cancer have been demonstrated in animals and humans with positive effects indicating a reduction in cancer cells, and even in some cases, the reversal of oral cancer.

- **Diabetes and Blood Sugar Improvement**

    A study from the University of Baroda in India revealed that spirulina may help diabetics. Over the course of a two-month study, patients with type 2 diabetes who were given two grams of spirulina every day improved blood sugar and lipid levels.

- **Immune System Boost**

    Tests on animals and senior citizens have exhibited a boost of the immune system, which is crucial to preventing viral infections. In these studies, spirulina was shown to increase the production of antibodies, which are needed to fight viral and bacterial infections, as well as some chronic illnesses.

- **Anti-Virus**

    Not only has the algae been observed to boos antibodies, but it has also shown an ability to hinder the replication of viruses. The National Cancer Institute (NCI) publicized that spirulina was "remarkably active" against the AIDS virus (HIV-1) after conducting a study in 1989. Test tube experiments have also shown spirulina to inhibit the replication of other viruses, including influenza A, mumps, and measles.

- **Antihistamine**

    In several scientific studies, spirulina appeared to help allergy symptoms such as watery eyes, skin reactions, and runny nose. In a recent study, a group of people suffering from rhinitis, an inflammation of the nasal mucous membrane, saw significant improvements of their allergy symptoms when given a daily 1000 mg or

2000 mg doses of spirulina over the course of twelve weeks.

- **Blood Pressure Reduction**

    Participants in an experiment at the National Autonomous University of Mexico were able to drop their blood pressure after taking spirulina for six weeks, without any other changes in their diet. Spirulina increases the body's production of nitric oxide, which is a gas that can widen blood vessels. Widened blood vessels improve the body's flow of blood, and ultimately can reduce blood pressure.

- **Lower Cholesterol**

    Recent research conducted in Greek universities has shown some promising effects on adults with high cholesterol. Over the course of three months, fifty-two adults were given one gram of spirulina each day. At the end of the three-month study period, the group's average triglycerides decreased over 16% and low-density lipoprotein (LDL) cholesterol (also known as the "bad" cholesterol) by 10%.

- **Radiation Treatment**

    After the Russian Chernobyl nuclear disaster in 1986, the Russian government turned to spirulina to treat children who had been exposed to the radiation.

Radiation destroys bone marrow, thus complicating the body's ability to create normal white or red blood cells. Within six weeks, children who were fed five grams of spirulina every day were able to make remarkable recoveries. The blue pigment of spirulina is comprised of phycocyanin, which enables the body to cleanse some radioactive metals.

- **Kidney and Liver Detoxification**

Not only has spirulina's phycocyanin been shown to cleanse radioactive metals, but it may also have the ability to cleanse heavy metal poisoning. Studies in Japan and elsewhere suggest that spirulina is able to safely assist in the removal of heavy metals such as arsenic, lead, mercury, and other similar metals that can be found in medicine, dental fillings, fish, deodorants, cigarettes, and drinking water.

- **Reducing Malnutrition**

According to the United Nations Food and Agricultural Organization, over 800 million people worldwide suffer from chronic undernourishment. Malnutrition is an epidemic as millions of people around the world lack enough proteins and micronutrients such as vitamins and minerals. With spirulina containing a significant amount of protein, B-vitamins, and iron, one tablespoon a day could eliminate micronutrient deficiencies that cause diseases such as anemia. Unlike other protein foods such as beef or nuts, spirulina is a very digestible source of protein. The digestive tract of malnourished individuals exhibits malabsorption, making the easily digestible spirulina, an even more attractive source of nourishment.

Chapter 13: Breakfast Recipes

1. Pancakes

Preparation time: 5 minutes

Cooking time: 15 minutes

Servings: 4

Ingredients:

- Egg – 1 large
- Egg whites – 2
- Cream cheese – 2 tbsp.
- Unsweetened, canned pumpkin – 3 tbsp. (not pie filling)
- Vanilla extract – 1 tbsp.
- Almond flour - 2/3 cup
- Coconut flour – 2 tbsp.
- Swerve sweetener – 1 tbsp.
- Pumpkin pie spice – 1 tsp
- Salt – 1/8 tsp

- Baking powder – 1 tsp
- Baking soda – ¼ tsp
- Xanthan gum – ½ tsp
- Water as needed

Topping:

- Cream cheese – 1/3 cup
- Unsweetened canned pumpkin – 2 tbsp.
- Swerve sweetener – 1 to 1 ½ tbsp.
- Cinnamon – ½ tsp
- Pumpkin pie spice – 1/8 tsp
- Vanilla extract – ½ tsp

Directions:

1. Preheat a griddle to 350°F and spray with non-stick cooking spray.
2. Add all the wet pancake ingredients except water into a blender and blend. Then add the dry ingredients and blend until smooth.
3. Add water a little at a time until the pancake batter has the right consistency.
4. Pour a small amount of batter onto a heated griddle.

5. Cook until browned and the edges (almost to the center) are dry about 3 to 4 minutes.

6. Then flip and cook for 2 to 3 minutes more.

7. For the topping: in a processor, add all topping ingredients and blend until creamy.

8. Top the pancakes with toppings and drizzle with maple syrup.

   Nutrition: Calories 206 Total Fat 14.4g Saturated Fat 7.5g Cholesterol 73mg Sodium 289mg Total Carbohydrate 11.1g Dietary Fiber 4.4g Total Sugars 1.4g Protein 7.6g.

2. Oatmeal

Preparation time: 5 minutes

Cooking time: 10 minutes

Servings: 6

Ingredients:

- Chia seeds - 1/3 cup
- Crushed pecans - 1 cup
- Cauliflower - 1/2 cup, riced
- Flaxseed meal - 1/3 cup
- Coconut milk - 3 1/2 cups
- Butter - 3 tbsp.
- Heavy cream - 1/4 cup
- Cream cheese - 3 oz.
- Maple flavor - 1 tsp
- Cinnamon - 1 1/2 tsp
- Erythritol - 3 tbsp. powdered
- Vanilla - 1/2 tsp
- Allspice - 1/4 tsp

- Nutmeg - 1/4 tsp

- Liquid stevia - 10-15 drops

- Xanthan gum - 1/8 tsp (optional)

Directions:

1. In a medium saucepan, heat milk over medium heat.

2. Crush pecans and add to the pan. Lower heat to toast.

3. Now add cauliflower to the coconut milk and bring to a boil. Reduce to simmer, add spices, and mix.

4. Grind erythritol and add to the pan. Then add chia seeds, flax, stevia and mix well.

5. Add butter, cream, and cream cheese to the pan and mix well.

6. Add xanthan gum to make it a bit thicker.

7. Serve.

Nutrition: Calories 485 Total Fat 46.5g Saturated Fat 22.5g Cholesterol 38mg Sodium 174mg Total Carbohydrate 21.7g Dietary Fiber 9.4g Total Sugars 10.7g Protein 7.7g.

3. Veggie Omelet

Preparation time: 5 minutes

Cooking time: 12 minutes

Servings: 1

Ingredients:

- Eggs – 3
- Almond milk or water – 1 tbsp.
- Kosher salt – ½ tsp
- Freshly ground black pepper – ½ tsp
- Unsalted butter – 3 tbsp.
- Swiss chard – 1 bunch, cleaned and stemmed
- Ricotta – 1/3 cup

Directions:

1. Crack the eggs in a bowl. Add water or milk, season with salt and pepper. Beat with a fork and set aside.
2. Melt 2 tbsp. butter over medium-high heat in an 8-inch nonstick skillet.
3. Add a few of the Swiss chard and continue to sauté until just wilted. Remove from pan. Set aside.

4. Melt 1 tbsp. butter in the skillet.

5. Then slowly add the egg mixture and tilt the pan, so the mixture spreads evenly. Allow the egg to firm up a bit. Cook for another 1 minute.

6. Spoon in the ricotta when the edges are firm, but the center is still a bit runny.

7. With a spatula, fold about 1/3 of the omelet over the ricotta filling.

8. Serve on a plate with Swiss chard.

Nutrition: Calories 652 Total Fat 57.9g Saturated Fat 33.2g Cholesterol 608mg Sodium 1776mg Total Carbohydrate 8.2g Dietary Fiber 1.2g Total Sugars 2.2g Protein 27.5g.

4. Ham Omelet

Preparation time: 5 minutes

Cooking time: 10 minutes

Servings: 5

Ingredients:

- Unsalted butter – 1 ½ tbsp.
- Eggs – 10
- Milk – 2 tbsp.
- Kosher salt – 1 tsp
- Freshly ground black pepper – ¼ tsp
- Cooked ham – 1 ¼ cups, diced
- Shredded sharp cheddar – 1 ½ cups
- Fresh chives – 1/3 cup, chopped

Directions:

1. Melt the butter in a skillet. Add ham and sauté until browned.
2. Meanwhile, whisk together the eggs, pepper, kosher salt, and milk in a bowl.

3. Pour into the pan and cook for 4 to 5 minutes, or until the desired doneness. Stirring occasionally.

4. Just before the eggs are set, add chives and cheddar.

Nutrition: Calories 175 Total Fat 9.4g Saturated Fat 5.1g Cholesterol 38mg Sodium 1084mg Total Carbohydrate 3.1g Dietary Fiber 0.6g Total Sugars 1g Protein 19g.

5. Low-Carb Cheese & Bacon Stuffed Meat Pies

Preparation Time: 10 mins

Cooking Time: 40 min

Servings: 4

Ingredient:

Filling:

- 500 g groundbeef (1.1 lb.)
- 4 large slices bacon, chopped (120 g/ 4.2 oz.)
- 1 small brown onion, chopped (g/ oz.)
- 1 tbsp coconut amines (15 ml)
- 2 tbsp tomato sauce/passata (30 ml)
- 1 cup beef stock or ban broth (240 ml/ 8 Fl oz)
- ½ tsp xanthan gum

Pie crust:

- 2 ¼ cups shredded mozzarella cheese (250g/8.8oz)
- 1 cup 2 tbsp shredded edam cheese (125g/4.4oz)
- 1/3 cup 1 tbsp full-fat cream cheese (100g/3.5oz)
- 1 ½ cups almond flour (150g/5.3oz)
- 2 large eggs

- 1 tsp onion powder
- 6 small chunks of sharp cheddar (66g/2.3oz)

Directions:

1. Cut the bacon into small strips and dice the onion.

2. Add to a skillet, along with the ground beef. Cook until just browned.

3. Add coconut aminos, passata, beef stock, and xanthan gum andstir well to combine. Bring to boil then reduce the heat and simmer for 30 minutes.

4. Remove from the heat and let cool. Once mixture is cool, heat oven to 200 °C/ 390 °F (fan assisted).

5. Prepare the pie crust. Place the cheeses and cream cheese into a large bowl and microwave for 1 minute. Remove and stir, then return for another 30 seconds. Repeat this once more. Add the almond meal, onion powder, and eggs and mix well until you have a soft dough.

6. Divide into four parts and sit one portion aside. Cut each of the remaining three portions in half and then flatten them out into large circles (you will have a total of six circles.)

7. Spray a six-hole oversized muffin pan and press the dough into cach cup, making sure to leave overhang at

the top as thedough will shrink while cooking. Bakefor 10 minutes.

8. Remove and spoon some filling into each cup. Press a chunk of cheddar intothecentre.

9. Then top with the remaining filling.

10. Divide the reserved dough into six and flatten out into lids. Lay the lid on top of the pies and gently press around the edges to seal. Cut a couple of steam vents in top of each pie.

11. Return to th eoven for 10-15 minutes until golden brown on top.

12. Ea twarm, with sugar-free ketchup if you want to feel very Australian. If you can't find sugar-free, you can make your own keto ketchup in just a few minutes!

13. Store in there frigerator for up to 5 days.

Nutrition: Net carbs: 2.3g Protein: 9.9g Fat: 8.2g Calories: 123kcal.

6. Avocado Egg Bowls

Preparation time: 5 minutes

Cooking time: 10 minutes

Servings: 3

Ingredients:

- 1 tsp coconut oil
- 2 organics, free-range
- Salt and pepper
- 1 Large & ripe avocado

For Garnishing:

- Chopped walnuts
- Balsamic Pearls
- Fresh thyme

Directions:

1. Slice your avocado in two, then take out the pit and remove enough of the inside so that there is enough space inside to accommodate an entire egg.

2. Cut off a little bit of the bottom of the avocado so that the avocado will sit upright as you place it on a stable surface.

3. Open your eggs and put each of the yolks in a separate bowl or container. Place the egg whites in the same small bowl. Sprinkle some pepper and salt to the whites, according to your personal taste, then mix them well.

4. Melt the coconut oil in a pan that has a lid that fits and put it on med-high.

5. Put in the avocado boats, with the meaty side down on the pan, the skin side up, and sauté them for approx. 35 seconds, or when they become darker in color.

6. Turn them over, then add to the spaces inside, almost filling the inside with the whites of the eggs.

7. Then, reduce the temperature and place the lid. Let them sit covered it for approx. 16 to 20 minutes until the whites are just about fully cooked.

8. Gently add one yolk onto each of the avocados and keep cooking them for 4 to 5 mins, just until they get to the point of cook you want them at.

9. Move the avocados to a dish and add toppings to each of them using the walnuts, the balsamic pearls, or/and thyme.

Nutrition: Calories 215 Fat 18g Carbohydrates 8g Protein 9g.

7. Chia Seed Banana Blueberry Delight

Preparation Time: 30 minutes

Cooking Time:

Servings: 2

Ingredients:

- 1 cup yogurt
- ½ cup blueberries
- 1/2 tsp Salt
- 1/2 tsp Cinnamon
- 1 banana
- 1 tsp Vanilla Extract
- 1/4 cup Chia Seeds

Directions:

1. Discard the skin of the banana.
2. Cut into semi-thick circles.
3. You can mash them or keep them as a whole if you like to bite into your fruits.
4. Clean the blueberries properly and rinse well.
5. Soak the chia seeds in water for 30 minutes or longer.

6. Drain the chia seeds and transfer them into a bowl.

7. Add the yogurt and mix well.

8. Add the salt, cinnamon, and vanilla and mix again.

9. Now fold in the bananas and blueberries gently.

10. If you want to add dried fruit or nuts, add it and then serve immediately.

11. This is best served cold.

Nutrition: Calories 260 Fats 26.6g Carbohydrates 17.4g Protein 4.1g.

8. Savory Breakfast Muffins

Preparation time: 10 minutes

Cooking time: 35 minutes

Servings: 6

Ingredients:

- 8 eggs
- 1 cup shredded cheese
- Salt and pepper to taste
- ½ tsp baking powder
- ¼ cup diced onion
- 2/3 cup coconut flour
- 1 ½ cup spinach
- ¼ cup full fat coconut milk
- 1 tbsp. basil, chopped
- ½ cup cooked chicken, diced finely

Directions:

1. Preheat the oven to 375-degree F.
2. Use butter or oil to grease your muffin tray or you can use muffin paper liners.

3. In a large mixing bowl, whisk the eggs.

4. Add in the coconut milk and mix again.

5. Gradually shift in the coconut flour with baking powder salt.

6. Add in the cooked chicken, onion, spinach, basil, and combine well.

7. Add the cheese and mix again.

8. Pour the mixture onto your muffin liners.

9. Bake for about 25 minutes.

10. Serve at room temperature.

Nutrition: Calories 388 Fat 25.8g Carbohydrate 8.6g Proteins 25.3g.

9. Morning Meatloaf

Preparation Time: 10 minutes

Cooking Time: 20 minutes

Servings: 6

Ingredients:

- 1 ½ pound of breakfast sausage
- 6 large organic eggs
- 2 tablespoons of unsweetened non-dairy milk
- 1 small onion, finely chopped
- 2 medium garlic cloves, peeled and minced
- 4-ounces of cream cheese softened and cubed
- 1 cup of shredded cheddar cheese
- 2 tablespoons of scallions, chopped
- 1 cup of water

Directions:

1. Add all the ingredients apart from water in a large bowl. Stir until well combined.
2. Form the sausage mixture into a meatloaf and wrap with a sheet of aluminum foil. Ensure that the meatloaf

fits inside your Instant Pot. If not, remove parts of the mixture and reserve for future use.

3. Once you wrap the meatloaf into a packet, add 1 cup of water and a trivet to your Instant Pot. Put the meatloaf on the trivet's top.

4. Cover and cook for 25 minutes on high pressure. When done, quickly release the pressure. Carefully remove the lid.

5. Unwrap the meatloaf and check if the meatloaf is done. Serve and enjoy!

Nutrition: Calories 592 Carbohydrates 2.5g Proteins 11g Fats 49.5g

10. Green Pineapple

Preparation Time: 5 minutes

Cooking Time: 0 minutes

Servings: 3

Ingredients:

- 1/2 of a pineapple
- 1 broccoli, diced
- 1 cup of water
- 1 long cucumber, diced
- A dash of salt
- 1 kiwi, diced

Directions:

1. Add kiwi, cucumber, pineapple, broccoli, and water in a blender.
2. Add the salt and blend until smooth.
3. Serve.

Nutrition: Calories 251 Fats 0.4g Proteins 0.5g Carbohydrates 22g .

Chapter 14: Lunch Recipes

11. Salmon with Sauce

Preparation time: 5 minutes

Cooking time: 15 minutes

Servings: 2

Ingredients

- Salmon fillet - 1 1/2 lb.
- Duck fat - 1 tbsp.
- Dried dill weed - ¾ to 1 tsp
- Dried tarragon - ¾ to 1 tsp
- Salt and pepper to taste
- Cream Sauce:
- Heavy cream - 1/4 cup
- Butter - 2 tbsp.
- Dried dill weed - 1/2 tsp
- Dried tarragon - 1/2 tsp
- Salt and pepper to taste

Directions:

1. Slice the salmon in half and make 2 fillets. Season skin side with salt and pepper and meat of the fish with spices.

2. In a skillet, heat 1 tbsp. duck fat over medium heat.

3. Add salmon to the hot pan, skin side down.

4. Cook the salmon for about 5 minutes. When the skin is crisp, lower the heat and flip salmon.

5. Cook salmon on low heat for 7 to 15 minutes or until your desired doneness is reached.

6. Remove salmon from the pan and set aside.

7. Add spices and butter to the pan and let brown. Once browned, add cream and mix.

8. Top salmon with sauce and serve.

Nutrition: Calories 449 Total Fat 34.5g Saturated Fat 14.4g Cholesterol 136mg Sodium 168mg Total Carbohydrate 1.1g Dietary Fiber 0.1g Total Sugars 0g Protein 35.2g.

12. Butter Chicken

Preparation time: 5 minutes

Cooking time: 30 minutes

Servings: 4

Ingredients:

- Butter – ¼ cup
- Mushrooms – 2 cups, sliced
- Chicken thighs – 4 large
- Onion powder – ½ tsp
- Garlic powder – ½ tsp
- Kosher salt – 1 tsp
- Black pepper – ¼ tsp
- Water – ½ cup
- Dijon mustard – 1 tsp
- Fresh tarragon – 1 tbsp., chopped

Directions:

1. Season the chicken thighs with onion powder, garlic powder, salt, and pepper.
2. In a sauté pan, melt 1 tbsp. butter.

3. Sear the chicken thighs about 3 to 4 minutes per side, or until both sides are golden brown. Remove the thighs from the pan.

4. Add the remaining 3 tbsp. of butter to the pan and melt.

5. Add the mushrooms and cook for 4 to 5 minutes or until golden brown. Stirring as little as possible.

6. Add the Dijon mustard and water to the pan. Stir to deglaze.

7. Place the chicken thighs back in the pan with the skin side up.

8. Cover and simmer for 15 minutes.

9. Stir in the fresh herbs. Let sit for 5 minutes and serve.

Nutrition: Calories 414 Total Fat 32.9g Saturated Fat 13.6g Cholesterol 149mg Sodium 786mg Total Carbohydrate 2g Dietary Fiber 0.5g Total Sugars 0.8g Protein 26.5g

13. Lamb Curry

Preparation time: 10 minutes

Cooking time: 4 hours

Servings: 6

Ingredients:

- Fresh ginger – 2 tbsp. grated
- Garlic – 2 cloves, peeled and minced
- Cardamom – 2 tsp
- Onion – 1 peeled and hopped
- Cloves – 6
- Lamb meat – 1 pound, cubed
- Cumin powder – 2 tsp
- Garam masala – 1 tsp
- Chili powder – ½ tsp
- Turmeric – 1 tsp
- Coriander – 2 tsp
- Spinach – 1 pound
- Canned – 14 ounces

Directions:

1. In a slow cooker, mix lamb with tomatoes, spinach, ginger, garlic, onion, cardamom, cloves, cumin, garam masala, chili, turmeric, and coriander.

2. Stir well. Cover and cook on high for 4 hours.

3. Uncover slow cooker, stir the chili, divide into bowls, and serve.

Nutrition: Calories 186 Total Fat 7.2g Saturated Fat 2.5g Cholesterol 38mg Sodium 477mg Total Carbohydrate 16.3g Dietary Fiber 5g Total Sugars 5g Protein 14.4g.

14. GarlicMushroom Frittata

Preparation time: 30 mins

Cooking time: 10 to 30 mins

Servings: 2

Ingredients:

- Low-calorie cooking spray
- 250g/9oz chestnut mushrooms, sliced
- 1 smallgarlicclove, crushed
- 1 tbsp. thinly slicedfresh chives
- 4 large free-range eggs, beaten
- freshlyground black pepper

For the Salad

- 1 LittleGem lettuce, leaves separated
- 100g/3½oz cherrytomatoes halved
- 1/3 cucumber, cut into chunks

Directions:

1. Spray a small, flame-proof frying pan with oil and place over a high heat. (The base of the pan shouldn't bewiderthanabout 18cm/7in.) Stir-fry the mushrooms

in threebatches for 2-3 minutes, or until softenedandlightlybrowned. Tip thecooked mushrooms into a sieveover a bowl tocatchanyjuices - youdon'twantthe mushrooms tobecome soggy.
2. Returnall the mushroomsto the pan and stir in thegarlic and chives, and a pinch of ground black pepper. Cookfor a further minute,thenreducethe heat tolow.
3. Preheatthe grill to its hottest setting. Pourtheeggsoverthemushrooms. Cookforfive minutes, or until almost set.
4. Placethepanunder the grill for 3-4 minutes, or until set.
5. Combine the salad ingredients in a bowl.
6. Remove fromthe grill andloosen the sides ofthefrittata with a round-bladed knife. Turn out onto a boardandcutintowedges. Servehotor cold with thesalad.

Nutrition: 243 kcal, 14g protein, 3.5g carbohydrate (ofwhich 3g sugars), 14g fat (of which 4g saturates), 2.5g fiberand 0.6g salt per portion

15. Salmon BLTs

Preparation Time: 0 mins

Cooking Time: 20 mins

Servings: 4

Ingredients:

- 8 slices bacon
- ½ c. low-fat Greek yogurt
- ¼ c. dill, chopped
- 1 scallion, finely chopped
- 1 tbsp. oil of choice
- 4 oz. skinlesssalmonfillet
- 1 tomato, sliced
- Romaine lettuce for serving
- Toasted bread forserving
- Salt and pepper

Directions:

1. Working in batches, cookbacon in a large skillet onmedium heat until crisp for 5 to 6 minutes; transferto a paper towel-lined plate.

2. Meanwhile, in a bowl, combine low-fat Greek yogurt, chopped dill, finely chopped scallion, and ¼ tsp each salt and pepper.

3. Wipe out the skillet and heat 1 Tbsp oil on medium. Season four 4-oz pieces of skinless salmon fillet with ¼ tsp each salt and pepper and cook until opaque throughout, 1 to 2 minutes per side.

4. Spread the yogurt mixture on 4 pieces of bread. Top with romaine lettuce, salmon, 1 sliced tomato, and bacon, then sandwich with another slice of bread.

Nutrition: 485 calories, 42g protein, 43g carbs, 7g fiber, 10g sugars (6g added sugars), 15g fat (4g sat fat), 72mg cholesterol, 885mg sodium.

16. Italian Style Meatballs with Courgette 'Tagliatelle'

Preparation time: 30 mins

Cookingtime: 10 to 30 mins

Servings: 2

Ingredients:

For the Meat Balls

- 250g/9oz extraleanbeefmince (5% fat or less)
- 1 small onion, veryfinelychopped
- 1 tspdried mixed herbs
- caloriecontrolledcookingoilspray
- 1 garlic clove, crushed
- 227g/8oz canchoppedtomatoes
- 2 heaped tbspfinelyshreddedfreshbasil leaves, plus extra to garnish

For theCcourgette 'Tagliatelle'

- 2 medium courgettes, trimmedanddeseeded
- Sea salt and freshly ground blackpepper

Directions:

1. Place the beef, half the onion, half the mixed herbs and a pinch of salt and pepper in a bowl and mix well. Form into 10 small balls.

2. Spray a medium non-stick fryingpan with a little oil and cook the meat balls for 5-7 minutes, turning occasionally until browned on allsides. Transferto a plate.

3. For the sauce, put the remaining onion in the same pan and cook over a low heat for three minutes, stirring. Add the garlic and cook for a few seconds.

4. Stir in the tomatoes, 300ml/10fl oz water, the remaining mixed herbs and shredded basil. Bring to the boil, stirring. Return the meatballs to the pan, reduce the heat to a simmer and cook for 20 minutes, stirring occasionally until the sauce is thick and the meatballs are cooked throughout.

5. Meanwhile, half-fill a medium pan with waterand bring tothe boil. Use a vegetable peeler to peel the courgettes into ribbons. Cook the courgette in th eboiling water for one minute then drain.

6. Divide the courgette ribbons between two plates and top with the meatballsand sauce. Garnish with basilleaves.

Nutrition: 219 kcal per portion.

17. Red Mullet with Baked Tomatoes

Preparation time: 30 mins

Cooking time: 10 to 30 mins

Servings: 4

Ingredients:

For the Tomatoes

- 375g/13oz mixedredandyellowcherrytomatoes
- 320g/11½oz finegreenbeans, trimmed
- 2 garliccloves, finelychopped
- 2 tbsp lemon juice
- Low-calorie cooking spray
- Salt and freshly ground blackpepper

For the Red Mullet

- 8 red mullet fillets, approximately 100g/3½oz each
- 1 lemon, finely grated rind only
- 2 tsp baby capers, drained
- 2 springonions, finelysliced

To Garnish

- 2 tbsp chopped parsley

- 8 caperberries

Directions:

1. Preheat the oven to 200C/180C Fan/Gas 6.

2. Put the tomatoes in an oven proof dish with the beans, garlic, lemon juice and spray with the oil. Season with salt and freshly ground black pepper and mix well. Bakefor 10 minutes, or until the tomatoes and beans aretender.

3. Meanwhile, tear off 4 large sheets of foil and line with non-stick baking paper. Place 2 fish fillets on each piece of baking paper, then scatter over the lemon rind, capers and spring onions, season with salt and freshly ground black pepper. Fold over the paper-lined foil and scrunch the edges together to seal. Placethe parcels on a large baking tray.

4. Place the fish parcels next to the vegetables in the oven and bake for a further 8-10 minutes, or until the flesh flakes easily when pressed in the centre with a knife.

5. Spoon the vegetables onto four serving plates and top each with two fish fillets. Garnish with the parsley and caper berries and serve.

Nutrition: 248 kcal.

18. Keto Crispy Ginger Mackerel Lunch Bowl

Preparation Time: 20 mins

Cooking Time: 15 mins

Servings: 2

Ingredients :

Marinade:

- 1 table spoon grated ginger
- 1 table spoon lemon juice
- 3 table spoons olive oil
- 1 table spoon coconut aminos
- Salt and pepper, totaste

Lunch bowl:

- 2 (8-ounce) bonelessmackerel fillets
- 1-ounce almonds
- 1 ½ cups broccoli
- 1 tablespoonbutter
- ½ smallyellow onion
- 1/3 cup diced red bell pepper
- 2 small sun-dried tomatoes, chopped

- 4 table spoons mashed avocado

Directions:

1. Preheat the oven to 400 °F. Line a baking tray with parchment paper or foil. Mix together the grated ginger, lemon juice, olive oil, coconut aminos, and some salt and pepper. Rub half of the marinade on the mackerel fillets.

2. Lay the fillets onto the baking tray with the skin side facing up. Roast for 12-15 minutes or until the skin is crispy.

3. Spread the almonds out on a separate baking sheet. Roastfor 5-6 minutes or until they brown. Take out of the oven and coo before chopping.

4. Lightly steam the broccoli until it'sstarted to soften but isn't mushy. Roughly chop it up.

5. Prehcat a pan over medium heat, then add the butter and allow it to melt. Fry the onions and peppers until they are soft.

6. Add the broccoli and sun-dried tomatoes, then continue cooking until warmed through.

7. Turn off the heat then mix in the rest of the dressing and roasted almonds. Serve with the avocado.

Nutrition: 649.55 Calories, 53.4g Fats, 9.2g Net Carbs, and 28.05g Protein

19. Zuppa Toscana with Cauliflower

Preparation time: 5 minutes

Cooking time: 25 minutes

Servings: 4

Ingredients:

- 1-pound ground Italian sausage
- 6 cups homemade low-sodium chicken stock
- 2 cups cauliflower florets - 1 onion, finely chopped
- 1 cup kale, stemmed and roughly chopped
- 1 (14.5-ounce) can of full-fat coconut milk
- ¼ teaspoon of sea salt
- ¼ teaspoon freshly cracked black pepper

Directions:

1. On the Instant Pot, press "Sauté" and add the ground Italian sausage. Cook until brown, stirring occasionally and breaking up the meat with a wooden spoon.
2. Add the remaining ingredients except for the kale and coconut milk and stir until well combined.
3. Cover and cook for 10 minutes on high pressure. When done, release the pressure naturally and remove the lid.

Stir in the kale and coconut milk. Cover and sit for 5 minutes or until the kale has **wilted. Serve and enjoy!**

Nutrition: Calories 653 Carbohydrates 8g Protein 26g Fat 4g.

20. Pork Carnitas

Preparation time: 20 minutes

Cooking time: 1 hour

Servings: 4

Ingredients:

- 6 medium garlic cloves, minced
- 2 teaspoons ground cumin
- 1 teaspoon smoked paprika
- 3 chipotle peppers in adobo sauce, minced
- 1 teaspoon dried oregano
- 2 bay leaves
- 1 cup homemade low-sodium chicken broth
- Fine sea salt and freshly cracked black pepper
- 2 tablespoons of olive oil
- 2 ½ pounds boneless pork shoulder, cut into 4 large pieces

Directions:

1. Season the pork shoulder with sea salt, black pepper, ground cumin, dried oregano, and smoked paprika.

2. On the Instant Pot, press "Sauté" and add the olive oil.

3. Once hot, add the pork pieces and sear for 4 minutes per side or until brown.

4. Add the remaining ingredients inside your Instant Pot. Cover and cook for 80 minutes on high pressure. When done, quick release the pressure and remove the lid.

5. Carefully shred the pork using two forks and continue to stir until well coated with the liquid.

6. Remove the bay leave and adjust the seasoning if necessary. Serve and enjoy!

Nutrition: Calories 170 Carbohydrates 2g Protein 4g Fat 8g.

Chapter 15: Snacks Recipes

21. Lamb and Flageolet Bean Stew

Preparation time: 30 mins

Cooking time: 1 to 2 hours

Servings: 4

Ingredients:

- 1 tsp olive oil
- 350g/12oz lean lamb, cubed
- 16 pickling onions
- 1 garlic clove, crushed
- 600ml/20fl ozlamb stock (made with concentrated liquid stock)
- 200g can of chopped tomatoes
- 1 bouquet garni
- 2 x 400g cans flageolet beans, drained and rinsed
- 320g/11oz green beans
- 250g/9oz cherry tomatoes

- Freshly ground blackpepper

Directions:

1. Heat the oil in a flameproof casseroleor saucepan, add the lamb and fry for 3-4 minutes until browned all over. Remove the lamb from the casserole and set aside.
2. Add the onions andgarlic to the pan and fry for 4-5 minutes, or until the onions are beginningto brown.
3. Return the lamband any juices to the pan. Add the stock, tomatoes, bouquet garni, and beans. Bring totheboil, stirring, then coverandsimmerfor 1 hour, or until the lamb is just tender.
4. Meanwhile, bring a panof water tothe boil andblanch the greenbeans. Place in a bowlof ice-cold water.
5. Add the cherry tomatoes tothe stew andseasonwell with freshly ground blackpepper. Continueto simmer for 10 minutes.
6. Dividethe stew betweenfourplates, place the greenbeansalongsideand serve.

Nutrition: 288 kcalperportion.

22. Chermoula Tofu and roasted Vegetables

Preparation time: 30 mins

Cooking time: 30 minsto 1 hour

Servings: 4

Ingredients:

For the Chermoula Tofu

- 25g/1oz coriander, finely chopped
- 3 garlic cloves, chopped
- 1 tsp cumin seeds, lightly crushed
- 1 lemon, finely grated rind
- ½ tspdried crushed chillies
- 1 tbsp olive oil
- 250g/9oz tofu

For the roasted Vegetables

- 2 redonions, quartered
- 2 courgettes, thickly sliced
- 2 red peppers, deseeded and sliced
- 2 yellow peppers, deseeded and sliced

- 1 small aubergine, thickly sliced
- Low-caloriecookingspray
- Pinch salt

Directions:

1. Preheat the oven to 200C/180C Fan/Gas 6.
2. For the chermoula, mix the coriander, garlic, cumin, lemon rind and chilies together with the oil and a little salt in a small bowl.
3. Pat the tofu dry on kitchen paper and cut it in half. Cut each half horizontally into thin slices. Spread the chermoula generously over the slices.
4. Scatter the vegetables in a roasting tin and spray with oil. Bake for about 45 minutes, until lightly browned, turning the ingredients once ortwice during cooking.
5. Arrange the tofu slices over the vegetables, with the side spread with the chermoula uppermost, and bake for a further 10-15 minutes, or until the tofu is lightly coloured.
6. Divide the tofu and vegetables between four plates and serve.

Nutrition: 182 kcal perportion.

23. Hearty Vegetable Soup

Preparation time: 30 mins

Cooking time: 30 mins to 1 hour

Servings: 2

Ingredients:

Calorie controlled Cooking Oil Spray

- 1 medium onion, sliced
- 2 garlic cloves, thinly sliced
- 2 celery sticks, trimmed and thinly sliced
- 2 medium carrots or 2 yellow peppers, cut into 2cm/1in chunks
- 400g/14oz tin chopped tomatoes
- 1 vegetable stock cube
- 1 tsp dried mixed herbs
- 400g/14oz tin butter beans, drained and rinsed
- 1 head young spring greens (approximately 125g/4½oz), trimmed and sliced
- Sea salt and freshly ground black pepper

Directions:

1. Spray a largenon-stick saucepan with oil and cook the onion, garlic, celery and carrots or peppers gently for 10 minutes, stirring regularly until softened.

2. Add 750ml/26fl oz water and the chopped tomatoes. Crumble over the stock cube and stir in the dried herbs. Bring to the boil, then reduce the heat to a simmer and cook for 20 minutes.

3. Season the soup with salt and pepper and add the spring greens and butter beans. Return to a gentle simmer and cook for a further 3-4 minutes or until the greens are softened. Season to taste and serve in deep bowls.

Nutrition: 219 kcalper portion.

24. Italian Omelet

Preparation Time: 10 mins

Cooking Time: 20 mins

Servings: 2

Ingredients:

For Topping

- 1 medium (½ cup) tomato, seeded, chopped

- 2 tables poons sliced green onion
- 1 tablespoon chopped fresh basil leaves

For Eggs

- 1 tables poon Land O Lakes® Butter
- 1 tea spoon finely chopped fresh garlic
- 4 large Land O Lakes® Eggs
- 1 table spoon water or milk
- ¼ tea spoonsalt
- 1/8 tea spoon pepper
- ½ cup shredded mozzarellacheese
- 2 table spoons shredded Parmesan cheese

Directions:

1. Combine all topping ingredients in bowl; set aside.
2. Melt butter in 10-inch nonstick skillet over medium heat until sizzling. Add garlic; cook 1 minute.
3. Beat eggs, water, salt and pepper in bowl at low speed until light in color and well mixed. Pour eggs into hot skillet. Cook 2 minutes; lift edge of eggs with heat proof spatula to allow uncooked portion to flow underneath 3-4 minutes or until mixture is almost set.

4. Sprinkle mozzarella cheese over half of omelet. Cover; let stand 1-2 minutes or until cheese is melted. Gently fold other half of omelet over cheese.

5. Place omelet onto plate; top with Parmesan cheese and tomato mixture. Cut in half.

Nutrition: 310 Calories 23Fat (g) 455 Cholesterol (mg) 720 Sodium (mg) 4 Carbohydrates (g) 1 Dietary Fiber 21 Protein (g).

25. Chocolate Truffles

Preparation time: 10 minutes

Cooking time: 60 minutes

Servings: 12

Ingredients:

- Ripe Hass avocados – 2 pitted and skinned
- Coconut oil – 2 tbsp.
- Premium cocoa powder – ½ cup
- Granulated sugar substitute – 1 tbsp.
- Sugar-free chocolate-flavored syrup – 2 tbsp.
- Heavy whipping cream – 2 tbsp.
- Bourbon – 2 tbsp.
- Chopped pecans – ½ cup

Directions:

1. Combine all ingredients except pecans in a small blender and process until smooth. Chill for 1 hour.
2. Make 1-inch balls and then roll in the pecans.
3. Chill in the refrigerator.

Nutrition: Calories 124 Total Fat 11.7g Saturated Fat 4g Cholesterol 3mg Sodium 9mg Total Carbohydrate 4.5g Dietary Fiber 2.9g Total Sugars 0.4g Protein 1.8g.

26. Blueberry Cake

Preparation time: 10 minutes

Cooking time: 40 minutes

Servings: 4

Ingredients:

- Almond flour – 2/3 cup
- Eggs – 5
- Almond milk – 1/3 cup
- Erythritol – ¼ cup
- Vanilla extract – 2 tsp
- Juice of 2 lemons
- Lemon zest – 1 tsp
- Baking soda – ½ tsp
- Pinch of salt
- Fresh blueberries – ½ cup
- Butter – 1 to 2 tbsp. melted

For the frosting:

- Heavy cream – ½ cup
- Juice of 1 lemon
- Erythritol – 1/8 cup

Directions:

27. Preheat the oven to 350°F.

28. In a bowl, add the almond flour, eggs, and almond milk and mix well until smooth.

29. Then add the erythritol, a pinch of salt, baking soda, lemon zest, lemon juice, and vanilla extract. Mix and combine well.

30. Fold in the blueberries.

31. Use the butter to grease the springform pans.

32. Pour the batter into the two greased pans.

33. Place on a baking sheet for even baking.

34. Place in the oven to bake until cooked through in the middle and slightly brown on the top about 35 to 40 minutes.

35. Allow cooling before removing from the pan.

36. Mix together the erythritol, lemon juice, heavy cream for the frosting. Mix well.

37. Pour frosting on top and spread. Serve.

Nutrition: Calories 272 Total Fat 23.8g Saturated Fat 13.2g Cholesterol 240mg Sodium 287mg Total Carbohydrate 21g Dietary Fiber 1.4g Total Sugars 18.2g Protein 8.9g.

27. Low-Carb Brownies

Preparation time: 10 minutes

Cooking time: 20 minutes

Servings: 16

Ingredients:

- 7 tablespoons Coconut oil, melted
- 6 tablespoons Plant-Based sweetener
- 1 Large egg
- 2 Egg yolk
- 1/2 tsp Mint extract
- 5 ounces Sugar-free dark chocolate
- ¼ cup Plant-based chocolate protein powder
- 1 tsp Baking soda
- ¼ tsp Sea salt
- 2 tablespoons vanilla almond milk, unsweetened

Directions:

1. Start by preheating the oven to 350°F and then take an 8x8 inch pan and line it with parchment paper, being

sure to leave some extra sticking up to use later to help you get them out of the pan after they are cooked.

2. Into a medium-sized vessel, use a hand mixer, and blend 5 Tablespoons of the coconut oil (save the rest for later), as well as the egg, Erythritol, egg yolks, and the mint extract all together for 1 minute. After this minute, the mixture will become a lighter yellow hue.

3. Take 4 oz of the chocolate and put it in a (microwave-safe) bowl, as well as with the other 2 Tablespoons of melted coconut oil.

4. Cook this chocolate and oil mixture on half power, at 30-second intervals, being sure to stir at each interval, just until the chocolate becomes melted and smooth

5. While the egg mixture is being beaten, add in the melted chocolate mixture into the egg mixture until this becomes thick and homogenous.

6. Add in your protein powder of choice, salt, baking soda, and stir until homogenous. Then, vigorously whisk your almond milk in until the batter becomes a bit smoother.

7. Finely chop the rest of your chocolate and stir these bits of chocolate into the batter you have made.

8. Spread the batter evenly into the pan you have prepared, and bake this until the edges of the batter just begin to become darker, and the center of the batter rises a little bit. You can also tell by sliding a toothpick into the middle, and when it comes out clean, it is ready. This will take approximately 20 to 21 minutes. Be sure that you do NOT over bake them!

9. Let them cool in the pan they cooked in for about 20 minutes. Then, carefully use the excess paper handles to take the brownies out of the pan and put them onto a wire cooling rack.

10. Make sure that they cool completely, and when they do, cut them, and they are ready to eat!

Nutrition: Calories 107 Fats 10g Carbohydrates 5.7g Protein 2.5g.

28. Apple Bread

Preparation time: 10 minutes

Cooking time: 20 minutes

Servings: 10

Ingredients:

- ½ cup honey
- ½ tsp. nutmeg
- ½ tsp. salt
- 1 cup applesauce, sweetened
- 1 tsp. baking soda
- 1 tsp. vanilla extract
- 2 ¼ cup whole wheat flour
- 2 large eggs
- 2 tbsp. vegetable oil
- 2 tsp. baking powder
- 2 tsp. cinnamon
- 4 cup apples, diced

Directions:

1. Preheat oven to 375° Fahrenheit and oil a loaf pan with non-stick spray or your choice of oil.

2. Beat eggs in a mixing bowl and stir until completely smooth.

3. Add the honey, oil, applesauce, cinnamon, vanilla, nutmeg, baking powder, baking soda, and salt. Whisk until completely combined and smooth.

4. Add the flour into the bowl and whisk to combine, making sure not to over-mix. Simply stir it enough to incorporate the flour.

5. Add apples to the batter and mix once more to combine.

6. Pour the batter into the loaf pan and smooth the top with your spatula.

7. Bake for 60 minutes, or until an inserted toothpick in the center comes out clean.

8. Let stand for 10 minutes, then transfer the loaf to a cooling rack to cool completely.

9. Slice into 10 pieces and serve!

Nutrition: Calories 210 Carbohydrates 41g Fats 5g Protein 5g.

29. Coconut Protein Balls

Preparation time: 20 minutes

Cooking time: 0 minutes

Servings: 27

Ingredients:

- ¼ cup of dark chocolate chips
- ½ cup coconut flakes, unsweetened
- ½ cup water
- 1 ½ cup almonds, raw & unsalted
- 2 tbsp. cocoa powder, unsweetened
- 3 cup Medjool dates, pitted
- 4 scoops whey protein powder, unsweetened

Directions:

1. Blend almonds in a food processor until a flour is formed. Add the water and dates to the flour and continue to process until fully combined. You may need to stop intermittently to scrape down the sides of the bowl.

2. Add cocoa and protein to the processor and continue to process until well combined. You may need to stop intermittently to scrape down the sides of the bowl.

3. Pull the blade out of the processor (carefully!) and use your spatula to gather all of the dough in one place inside the processor container.

4. On a plate or in a large, shallow dish, spread the coconut flakes.

5. Scoop out a little bit of the dough at a time using a spoon, and roll it into balls, then roll each one in the coconut flakes.

6. Refrigerate for at least 30 min before enjoying.

Nutrition: Calories 108 Carbohydrates 16g Fats 4g Protein 5g.

30. Chocolate Chia Pudding

Preparation time: 3 minutes

Cooking time: 0 minutes

Servings: 1

Ingredients:

- ¾ cup milk, unsweetened
- 2 tsp. honey
- 1 tsp. vanilla extract
- 4 tbsp. chia seeds
- 1 tbsp. cocoa powder, unsweetened

Directions:

1. In a glass jar or container, combine all liquid ingredients and mix completely.
2. Add chia seeds and cocoa powder and mix completely.
3. Allow everything to sit for about 10 minutes before stirring once again, then sealing tightly and storing it in the refrigerator overnight.
4. Stir well before eating and enjoy cold!

Nutrition: Calories 329 Carbohydrates 40g Fats 14g Protein 14g

Conclusion

In anything new that we try, there is a chance that we may fall off track. Fasting or following a new diet plan is no different. The focus should not be on the fact that you fell off but on how you decide to come back and approach it again. You need not give up altogether if you have a day or two where you did not accomplish your full fast. You just need to re-examine your plan and approach it in a different way. Maybe your fasting period was too long for your first try. Maybe your fasting and eating windows did not match up with your sleep-wake cycle as well as they could have. Any of these factors can be adjusted to better suit your lifestyle needs and make fasting or a specific diet work for you. Being able to be flexible with yourself is something that is trying a new diet regimen as this can teach you. With the human body, there is never a right or a wrong way to approach anything; there is only a multitude of different ways and some that will be better for your specific body and mind than others. Being open to trying different variations and adjusting your plan as you go can be the difference between success and decided to give up.

Intermittent fasting can be very challenging at first but if you can get over the few times and stick to it, it is immensely rewarding.

Don't give up if you feel that the fasting plan you have chosen is too much for you. Ask your medical advisor to help you either modify your current plan or try another one. Not everyone is suited to each plan. You may find you need to try one or two before you are comfortable.

If you fall off track, scale your plan back a little bit and try it again. If you are worried that you are not doing enough, begin with the scaled-back plan, and get used to this first, you can always increase your fasting times later on once you know you are completely comfortable with a shorter fasting time.

If this book has taught you anything, the hope is that it has taught you how many variables are involved when it comes to health and wellness. This book aimed to share with you the plethora of options that are available to you when it comes to autophagy and inducing it within the cells of your body.

Think back on the many options that were laid out for you involving diet options and specific foods that have the ability to induce autophagy in the brain. It is your job now to decide which of these foods or supplements to include in your life and to practice a sort of trial and error, noting which ones make you feel great and which ones you prefer to go without. With all of this information, you can decide which ways fit best with your specific lifestyle and your preferences.

As you take all of this information forth with you, it may seem overwhelming to begin applying this into your own life.

Remember, life is a process, and you do not need to expect perfection from yourself. By taking steps to read this book, you are already on your way to changing your life.

DASH DIET FOR WOMEN OVER 50

THE BEST NATURAL SOLUTION TO INTERVENE ON HIGH BLOOD PRESSURE. FOOD TIPS TO KEEP THE ARTERIES YOUNG AND RECIPES TO LOSE WEIGHT AND PROMOTE CARDIOVASCULAR WELL-BEING

Author: Keli Bay

Introduction

The DASH Diet is intended to help people who suffer from high blood pressure levels. By modifying your dietary patterns and choices to consuming delicious yet healthy food, you can keep your blood pressure levels in check. Aside from reducing your sodium intake, the DASH Diet also increases your absorption of Potassium, Magnesium, and Calcium. By following this diet, you will experience a drop in your blood pressure levels to a few points. And if you continually follow this diet regimen, your systolic blood pressure can go down by at the most 8 to 14 points.

DASH Diet and Weight Loss

Because the Dash Diet encourages you to consume only healthy foods, you will reduce your weight over a long time. It encourages you to consume complex carbohydrates and healthy starches. The complex carbohydrates contain plant materials such as cellulose and fiber that are not digested. They only bulk up on your stomach, making you feel full for a longer time. It will prevent you from craving too much, and since you are consuming foods that are caloric-dense, giving your body sufficient time to metabolize the food and use it as a source of energy.

DASH Diet Leads to A Healthier Kidney

The National Kidney Foundation supports the diet. Hypertension has a connection to kidney diseases. It also helps decrease the blood pressure level, more likely, reducing kidney diseases. A person has to limit his intake of salt, and other Sodium-rich foods can help reduce the formation of kidney stones.

Why DASH Diet Works?

Food plays a vital role in the development of hypertension. Researches have shown that consumption of foods rich in Sodium (salt), mainly processed food, can increase the likelihood of developing hypertension. But can diet alone help stabilize blood pressure levels? Researchers from the NIH noted that dietary interventions play vital roles in improving people suffering from different situations. Dietary change can decrease the systolic blood pressure level by about 6 to 11 mmHg. This means that following the right diet regimen and omitting foods that are not helpful to the blood pressure level can bring relief to hypertensive people.

The DASH Diet was developed by expert nutritionists and has undergone several trials to prove that it can benefit by reducing the systolic pressure. The reduction of the systolic blood pressure was observed not only among hypertensive individuals but also among those who have normal blood pressure levels.

Tips for Planning Your Dash Diet

The DASH Diet is one of the easiest ways to maintain a healthy lifestyle. When planning to do the DASH Diet, there are some things that you need to consider first. Below are essential tips for planning your DASH Diet.

• Make small changes: Remember that this particular diet regimen encourages you to make diet changes by eating whole foods. Making small changes allow you to adjust to this regimen easily. You can do this by gradually making changes in your diet. For instance, you can add more serving of vegetables every meal or substitute unhealthy dressings with healthier condiments.

• Limit your intake of meat: Start limiting the amount of meat that you are going to take in. If you are currently eating large amounts of meat, you can start cutting back at least two servings every day.

• Start avoiding full-fat options: Start avoiding full-fat options once you start planning to do the DASH Diet. It is easier to omit foods that are not allowed for this particular diet, especially when you began restricting yourself earlier in the first place.

- Start cooking healthy: When you cook your food, try learning how to cook without too much or no salt at all. This may be challenging for you, but you can try experimenting with different salt-free flavorings, herbs, and spices.

- Eat out less often: If you love to eat out all the time, try to minimize your dinner trips once you have started with the DASH Diet. This is especially true if you are still getting the hang of this diet. Most restaurants either use too much salt when flavoring their food. If you cannot help but eat out, ask the restaurant to prepare food without added salt or MSG.

- Plan your meals: Another tip to make you successful in your DASH Diet is to plan your meals. Preparing your meals weekly is a great way to stick to this diet. A weekly meal plan will also serve as your guide on when to eat and what to eat. This will help you avoid over-snacking or eating foods that you are not supposed to eat.

The Dash Diet Food Pyramid

The DASH Diet is a very straight-forward diet regimen, but it still helps, especially for starters like you, to have a guide. This is where the DASH Diet food pyramid comes in. The DASH Diet pyramid is just like your usual food guide, but it indicates what types of food you can eat for this particular diet regimen with specific serving amounts for a 2000-calorie daily diet.

The food pyramid is also carefully designed to reduce the total fat in food choices.

The food items that are listed at the bottom of the pyramid are the fruits and vegetables. They should be consumed at 8 to 10 servings daily. This is followed by whole grains. Both the low-fat and meats are at the third tier of the pyramid, which means you need to consume less of it. The fourth level of the pyramid includes beans, nuts, and seeds. At the same time, sweets belong to the top of the pyramid and should be taken with fewer servings weekly. If you notice, there are only three types of food groups included in the food pyramid.

Dash Diet Food No-Goes

With the DASH Diet, nothing is technically off-limits, but dieters are recommended to eat less of foods bad for the health. If you are new, you must know about which foods you should avoid and which foods to avoid.

• Red meat: Red meat is not recommended if you want to follow the DASH Diet. However, you can occasionally eat grass-fed beef as it is high in Omega-3 fatty acids due to its diet.

• Bad fats: As mentioned earlier, not all fats are created equally. Avoid bad fats, including margarine, hydrogenated vegetable oil, and vegetable shortening, because they promote atherogenesis.

• Salt or Sodium: The DASH Diet is a low salt diet or none at all, as salt can cause hypertension. Instead of using salt, use the spice rack to improve the flavor of your food.

• Alcohol: Consumption of alcohol can elevate your blood pressure levels. Too much alcohol can eventually damage the liver, brain, and heart. If you cannot avoid but drink alcohol, make sure that you drink one glass if you are a female and two if you are a man.

• Cured meats: All kinds of cured meats are not recommended because they contain high amounts of Sodium that may cause hypertension. Moreover, cured meats also contain potential carcinogens that can cause cancer.

• Full-fat dairy: The purpose of the DASH Diet is to lessen the intake of fat. This includes full-fat dairy, such as milk, cream, and cheese.

• Other foods: Other foods that are included in the no-eat list include high-fat snacks, sugary sweets or snacks, salad dressings, sauces, and gravies.

Chapter 16: Hypertension In Women: 5 Things To Know

Hypertension may cause heart disease and stroke. The following are the five things you have to know when it comes to Hypertension.

1. **Women Faces Higher Risk Than Men**

Males and females have a similar risk of developing high blood pressure in their 40s, 50s, and 60s. However, after the onset of menstruation, females are at greater risk of developing high blood pressure than men.

2. Hypertension can also happen to young people

In older people, high blood pressure doesn't happen spontaneously. one in five females ages 35 to 44 have hypertension.

It is also the leading cause of stroke, which also rises among younger individuals. Studies have shown that the increased risk for stroke is directly due to obesity, high blood pressure, as well as diabetes. Complications can be eliminated and treated. A younger individual should check their blood pressure at least once a year. To be aware of it, you have to check your blood pressure regularly as most with hypertension are not aware of it.

3. Hypertension doesn't display any symptoms

High blood pressure is often labeled as the "silent killer." there seem to be no signs, like sweating
or headaches, for most people with hypertension. They do not even think they need to have their
blood pressure checked since they feel fine.

4. Understanding Preeclampsia

When we say preeclampsia, this is a condition contributing to about 13 percent of all maternal deaths worldwide. It is generally a controllable complication, and after the infant is delivered, it usually goes away within two months. Most at risk are the following groups of females:

- Teenagers
- Females who have had multiple pregnancies
- Women in their 40
- Female who has a history of hypertension or kidney disease
- Females who are obese

5. Women Faces Unique Risks when it comes to hypertension

Ladies with hypertension who become pregnant are more likely than someone with normal blood pressure to have pregnancy complications. High blood pressure can harm the kidneys as well as other organs of a woman, causing early delivery and low birth weight. A woman can raise the risk of high blood pressure by using certain types of birth control.

Contraceptives and hypertension

The use of oral contraceptives typically increases the blood pressure by 8 mm Hg systolic and 6 mm Hg diastolic. Furthermore, depot medroxyprogesterone acetate does not significantly affect blood pressure. It also reported that it increases the risk of vascular events in women taking combination estrogen/progestin contraceptives. Due to it, the use of hormonal should be weighed against the risk of adverse pregnancy outcomes related to hypertension.

Those under 35 years, who controlled and monitored their hypertension well, are appropriate to take a test first if it is fine to take contraceptives with other medicines, especially If it shows no signs of end-organ vascular disease. If blood pressure remains controlled for months after the test is started, it may be continued. The appropriate options in women with hypertension are the levonorgestrel-releasing intrauterine system (Mirena) and progestin-only contraceptives.

Chapter 17: Symptoms Of Hypertension In Women

Sadly, most people don't have control with regard to their hypertension. This indicates a higher risk of hypertension complications and dangers, but all hope is not lost for you. Monitoring your numbers and taking the medications prescribed by your doctor is an excellent way to go.

Hypertension is when the blood pressure in your vessel is higher than usual. It is measured as the force of blood against your blood vessel walls, usually the arteries. And it is the actress that carries oxygenated blood to your tissues and the other organs in your body.

To know the symptoms of hypertension, you should first check your blood pressure. The blood pressure is measured with blood pressure tools, and the readings appear as one number over the other. The top number indicated is the systolic blood pressure number, and that is the force due to the contraction of your heart and when your heart pushes blood through your body. The number below is referred to as diastolic blood pressure number, and this force occurs when your heart relaxes—the classification of high blood pressure and normal blood pressure.

1. Normal blood pressure
- 90/60 - under 120/80 mm Hg
2. Risk of hypertension or prehypertension.
- 120-139/80-89 mm Hg
3. Stage 1 hypertension
- 140-159/90-99 mm Hg
4. Stage 2 hypertension
- Above 160/100 mm Hg

When your diastolic and systolic blood pressure appears on two different levels, your doctor will generally consider it at a higher level. An example is when your blood pressure reading is 135/91. This reading shows that your systolic blood pressure is in the prehypertension range, while in the stage 1 hypertension range is your diastolic blood pressure. This blood pressure reading of 135/91 will put you in the stage 1 hypertension category.

Symptoms Of Hypertension In Women

- Tiredness
- Loss of Energy
- Sleeping Disturbances
- Tight, nagging, and often continuous chest pain at rest

- Palpitations, tachycardias, paroxysmal atrial fibrillations
- Headaches, blurred vision
- Intermittent fluid retention, ankles, hands, and eyes

hypertension.

What can trigger essential high blood pressure?

Essential hypertension can also be referred to as primary high blood pressure.

More than 9 out of 10 cases of hypertension are essential. Essential hypertension is what people referred to as high blood pressure or hypertension. This type of hypertension is caused by direct factors such as genetic factors on lifestyle choices. The lifestyle choices that can cause essential hypertension include

- Obesity or being overweight.
- Smoking
- Lack of exercise or redundant lifestyle.
- Inadequate sleep.
- Stress
- Poor eating habits and eating high sodium diets

Secondary high blood pressure is another type of hypertension. Secondary hypertension is caused primarily by medical causes such as

- Adrenal disease
- Kidney disease
- Harmful medications such as over the counter oral contraceptives and painkillers

You should be aware of the risk factors of high blood pressure to be proactive in managing the condition. The risk factors associated with blood pressure are divided into two, and they are:

Non-Modifiable Risk Factors

The non-modifiable risk factor associated with high blood pressure are those factors you cannot control; they include.

- Family or genetic history: you have a higher risk of having hypertension if someone in your family, your siblings, or your parents have it.
- Age: It is one of the non-modifiable factors. As you age, the risk of you having high blood pressure increases
- Race: research has shown that black Americans or blacks, in general, are more at risk of having high blood pressure or the complication arising from it.

Modifiable risk factors

These factors are factors that can cause high blood pressure you can control. Knowing about these modifiable risk factors will help you adapt your life to prevent high blood pressure or regulate it.

Some of the modifiable risk factors include.

- Obesity: being overweight requires additional blood volume to carry oxygen to the tissues in your body. You are thereby leading your blood vessels to have extra pressure.

- Redundant lifestyle and lack of activity: lack of exercise will make your heart work extra hard to pump blood, causing extra pressure on your arteries.

- Smoking and tobacco consumption: tobacco and smoking can damage your arteries and increase your blood pressure.

- Eating high sodium and low potassium foods: foods with high sodium concentration increases your blood pressure while foods with potassium reduce your blood pressure.

- Excess alcohol intake: low intake of red wine might be right for your health, but excess consumption of alcoholic beverages will increase your blood pressure.

Chapter 18: How To Fight Hypertension

To fight Hypertension, you need to be mindful of what you eat and your activities. Below is the sample of a healthy lifestyle:

- Eating a healthy diet
- Maintaining a healthy weight
- Getting enough physical activity
- Not smoking
- Limiting alcohol use

You also need to keep away from the food the isn't good for health, such as

- Alcohol.
- Food trash: fast food, chocolate bars, chips. They only harm the body.
- Fatty foods (it also includes dairy products with high-fat content)
- All sodas, sweet and savory
- Canned meat and fish
- Pickles.
- Smoked products.
- Semi-finished products

- Sweets (only harmless sweets are allowed in minimal quantities: marshmallows, salads from sweet fruits, marshmallows)
- Baking, confectionery
- Salt and sugar (at first, their amount is gradually limited, then these products are excluded altogether).
- Hot spices.
- Coconut and palm vegetable oils.

Such a "blacklist" is typical for any diet that is considered healthy.

Healing Foods

Hypertension occurs when the sodium/potassium ratio becomes imbalanced due to a low potassium diet or a magnesium deficiency.

The average diet delivers too much sodium and too little potassium. Eating to reverse this imbalance could lower high blood pressure and reduce the risk of heart attack and stroke.

Minerals

A study found that a diet that includes plenty of foods rich in magnesium and potassium can help to control blood pressure, even without reducing sodium intake.

Foods rich in potassium are essential in managing hypertension as the potassium lessens the effects of sodium.

The more potassium you eat, the more sodium you lose through urine. Foods highest in potassium include lima beans, kale, avocado, spinach, salmon, and banana. Four thousand seven hundred milligrams (mg) per day are recommended potassium intake for an average adult.

Dark leafy greens, nuts, seeds, fish, beans, whole grains, avocados, yogurt, and bananas are included in high Magnesium foods. This recommends that you have to take 370 mg of magnesium citrate per day if you have hypertension.

Himalayan Salt

The body does need sodium in moderation from a healthy source like Himalayan salt. A study found 3 g per day is an estimated sodium intake between and 6g per day can lower the risk of death and cardiovascular events.

The Himalayan salt contains minerals that are good for maintaining health, including macrominerals and trace minerals.

Low-Gi Foods

The most common underlying cause of hypertension is high insulin levels. As insulin levels rise, it causes blood pressure to increase. Research shows that those who were insulin resistant also have high blood pressure.3 Lowering blood sugar levels will help lower blood pressure.

Foods with a high GI make a person's blood sugar levels rise rapidly, increasing their chance of getting diabetes. They also make managing type 2 diabetes a challenge. Foods with a low GI release glucose more slowly and steadily into the bloodstream and therefore have the most inadequate insulin response.

If blood sugar rises too quickly, the pancreas secretes a more significant amount of insulin. Insulin helps bring sugar out of the bloodstream, primarily by converting the excess sugar to stored fat. High blood sugar leads to more significant insulin release and more storage of fat.

Replace all white sugar and artificial sweeteners with the natural sweetener Stevia. It has a GI of zero, which means it does not raise blood sugar levels. Unlike sugar, which negatively affects insulin resistance, stevia has been shown to impact those with diabetes positively. Studies have found that stevia improves insulin sensitivity.

Eat Breakfast

Skipping breakfast or eating late at night causes weight gain and leads to higher fasting insulin, total cholesterol, and LDL cholesterol. You are better able to metabolize food during the day when you are awake and active. Food eaten right before bedtime or during the night will likely be converted into fat. A good breakfast consists of high potassium and high magnesium foods such as avocado toast with a kefir glass to drink.

Healing Supplements

Various types of complementary and alternative treatments are believed to be useful for treating high blood pressure.

Magnesium

Magnesium deficiency is a factor that leads to high blood pressure. Eighty percent of the population is the estimation of deficiency in vital mineral, according to health experts and nutritionists.

It has proven that magnesium supplementation treats hypertension. Fifteen mmol per day will lower blood pressure in patients treated with anti-hypertensive medications.8

Chromium

Chromium also plays a vital role in glucose metabolism, and there is evidence that it may help prevent insulin resistance. Chromium polynicotinate has been shown to reduce systolic blood pressure in those with high blood sugar.

Red Yeast Extract

Red Yeast Extract contains monacolin K, which has properties very similar to lovastatin. Red yeast rice may be beneficial in treating hypertension. It lowers cholesterol levels successfully.

Healthy Restaurant Choices

You can order heart-healthy options at any restaurant; you just have to be strategic. Here are some ordering tips to use when eating out:

- Request that your food is prepared without salt or salty seasonings.
- Keep condiments on the side.
- Watch your liquid calories and choose water as your beverage.
- Choose baked, broiled, and grilled entrées and skip the fried.
- Skip heavy cream sauces and prefer marinara over Alfredo-type spices.
- Go for fish, chicken, and vegetarian dishes instead of red meat.
- Watch portion sizes and fills half your plate with vegetables.
- Go easy on the bread and chips.

Healthy Mexican tips and picks:

Limit your intake of chips and start with tortilla soup instead. Opt for the vegetable- and bean-filled soft tacos, tamales, and burritos over fried items. Fajitas are the right choice because you can control the portions since the meat, veggies, toppings, and tortillas are all served separately.

Healthy Chinese tips and picks:

Skip the soup and noodles, and choose steamed dishes with sauce on the side. Choose entrées that come with a lot of vegetables like Moo Goo Gai Pan. Ask for brown rice instead of white.

Chapter 19: Health Self Assessment

Learn about high blood pressure by taking this quiz. Answer the questions and find out if you know how to keep fit and healthy.

1. Are you allowed to drink coffee or tea every day? Is it okay for your blood pressure?
2. Is weight exercise allowed when you have hypertension?
3. Can I weight heavy things?
4. Should you avoid licorice?
5. Is the sauna taboo?
6. Do you need to limit the consumption of salt if you have hypertension?

All of the answers would be discussed later on if you answered correctly, then, congratulations! You know how to keep yourself healthy, especially in lowering your blood pressure. If you answered no, then you have to read carefully and follow these simple tips.

High Blood Pressure: What Am I Allowed To Do And What Not?

If you have high blood pressure, you ask yourself many questions: Is coffee allowed? Do I have to do without the sauna? What about exercise? Our experts provide answers. If the doctor determines that you have high blood pressure, you will likely have numerous questions on your mind. The medic must have pointed out all sorts of things to you.

Nevertheless, new uncertainties arise frequently: Can I drink my beloved latte macchiato? What did the doctor say again about salt? We have picked up a few points for you:

Can I Drink Coffee Or Tea?

Usually: yes. However, coffee can and tea can temporarily raise blood pressure. But if you regularly drink a cup, the increase is lower and usually does not cause any problems. Then experts consider four to five cups a day to be acceptable. However, Dr. Heribert Brück, a cardiologist from Erkelenz and press spokesman for the Federal Association of Resident Cardiologists, said: "If you rarely drink coffee, your blood pressure can skyrocket by up to 20 mmHg." How much of the aromatic drink can be consumed varies significantly from person-person. Professor Hans-Georg Predel, a sports medicine specialist and high blood pressure expert from Hamburg, advises: "Measure your blood pressure after you've had coffee, then you will get a feel for how you react to it.

High Blood Pressure: Symptoms, Causes, Treatment

What do I have to consider when doing sports? Are weight exercises allowed?

In most cases, physical activity is permitted and makes sense. Because exercise can lower blood pressure in the long term - how pronounced this effect varies from person to person. "Endurance sports, in particular, have a positive effect," says Brück. These include, for example, cycling and walking. Doctors tend to advise against sports such as tennis or badminton because they have high-stress peaks.

Strength training can also have positive effects, although high-pressure patients should be careful with it. It is crucial here that you perform suitable exercises correctly, that you do not overtax yourself and that you seek advice on what weight you are allowed to lift. Therefore, the individual suitability and resilience should be clarified with the doctor, especially with strength training. The training should then take place under expert guidance and adapted to the particular situation.

Predel generally recommends high blood pressure patients who want to do sport: "Discuss with your doctor how intensively you can exercise yourself, have yourself examined by sports medicine and, if possible, exercise under supervision." Also important: If you have very high blood pressure values, you may not be allowed to do sports. Therefore, it is essential to clarify this beforehand - your treating doctor will provide you with information.

Can I lift heavy things?

This is - depending on the weight, among other things - not always prohibited—people whose artery is diseased need to be particularly careful. With them, the rise in blood pressure that results from the increased effort can quickly become dangerous. "This is especially true if you hold your breath or press it out while you breathe," said Predel.

Should I avoid licorice?

No, you don't have to. But it would help if you didn't overeat licorice and not regularly. "The ingredients can cause water to accumulate in the body and have an unfavorable effect on blood pressure," explains heart specialist Brück. However, this effect is only noticeable if you consume an appropriate amount every day. Quantities under 50 grams are generally not considered to be a problem.

Is there any special diet for people with high blood pressure?

Experts like Brück and Predel recommend eating a Mediterranean diet. According to studies, the following applies: Whoever eats a lot of vegetables and fruit, eats little meat and instead eats more fish, replaces animal fats with plant-based ones, and consumes less low-fat dairy products can have a positive effect on blood pressure. This type of diet corresponds to the traditional Mediterranean diet.

Is the sauna taboo?

Not always. Cardiovascular diseases can, however, in some instances, speak against a visit to the sauna. You should, therefore, ask your doctor. "The heat in the sauna expands the blood vessels, which lowers blood pressure," explains Brück. This can increase the effects of antihypertensive agents. Both blood pressure specialists also emphasize Cooldown carefully after the sauna! Do not jump into the cold plunge pool. Because the cold stimulus causes the blood vessels to contract and the blood pressure increases significantly. If the said temperature is cold enough, it is enough to briefly go into the cold air - until you feel the first chill. For example, experts advise against using the sauna if you have a cold with a fever that has recently had a heart attack or stroke, or your blood pressure significantly increased despite treatment. Also, watch out for dizziness in the sauna. The tension in the vessels may drop too much. Then leave the heated cabin, lie down, and rest.

Do I have to limit my salt consumption?

Medical professionals recommend that high blood pressure patients eat no more than six grams of salt a day. That's about a teaspoon because some of the patients react sensitively to excessively large quantities - the pressure in the vessels increases. "Even if not everyone benefits from not using salt, everyone should still try," advises Brück. Most of the salt does not come from the salt shaker, but certain foods. Bread, hard cheese, and sausage products such as ham or salami, for example, are full of salt. Frozen foods and canned foods are also often high in them.

Should I avoid alcohol?

Only drink alcohol in moderation - or do without it entirely. "If you consume alcohol regularly, your blood pressure can increase over time," says Brück. Predel adds: "Among other things, the stimulant has the effect of releasing stress hormones and messenger substances that increase blood pressure." Besides, the drink contains almost as many calories as fat and can thus promote obesity. It raises the risk of high blood pressure. If you keep the necessary amount, alcohol usually has little effect on the vessels' pressure: men can have two drinks a day, women one. But don't drink wine, beer, or brandy every day.

Chapter 20: Food Remedies That Protect The Arteries

Grains

Recommended servings: 6-8 per day

Grains are a foundational necessity of the DASH Diet due to their high fiber and low-fat content and nutrient density. However, for this to apply, the grains you consume need to be as whole and unrefined as possible. When choosing grains at the store, be careful when selecting products based on the words "whole grain" or "natural" alone. Products should indicate that they are one hundred percent whole grain, or the ingredient list should not have any refined or processed grain foods or refined sugars. We often add grains to our diets but tend to enhance them with heavy sauces or spreads. If this is you, it may take some time, but learn to appreciate the earthy nuttiness of pure whole grains without all of the added salty and fatty accompaniments.

One serving of grain would be one slice of whole wheat bread, ½ cup brown rice, ½ cup whole grain pasta, ½ cup of cooked oatmeal (or other hot grain cereal), approximately one ounce of dry whole-grain cereal.

Vegetables

Recommended servings: 4-5 per day

While following the DASH Diet, you will get most of your vital vitamins and nutrients through the produce, mainly vegetables, which you consume. The best vegetable choices for the DASH Diet are high in fiber, magnesium, potassium, and other vitamins. Most people today do not get anywhere near the recommended amount of vegetables in their diet, for several reasons. Vegetables are seen as a side dish and come in a small garden salad before dinner. Also, there is the misconception that vegetables are not convenient. They require cleaning, cooking, and seasoning to be considered palatable. This is simply not true, well except for the cleaning part. Vegetables are best when they are minimally prepared to bring out their fresh and unique flavors fully.

Begin to think of vegetables as more than just a side dish — instead, make them the center of at least one of your meals every day. Also, keep cleaned and chopped fresh vegetables on hand for easy and nutritious snacks.

One serving of vegetables equals ½ cup raw or cooked cut-up vegetables or 1 cup of uncooked leafy greens.

Fruits

Recommended servings: 4-5 per day

While not allowed during the short Phase One of the DASH Diet, in Phase Two, fresh fruit becomes a dietary necessity. Like vegetables, most fruit is high in fiber, potassium, and magnesium, and are low-fat and healthy ways to address a sweet craving. The great advantage of fresh fruit is that it requires little or no advanced preparation to be immediately edible, or you can dress it up in the form of an elegant new fruit dessert. Help get the recommended number of fruit servings in your diet by adding a piece of fresh fruit to the end of each meal and keep fruit on hand for a quick snack. You can also boost the fiber benefit of the fruits you eat by keeping on any edible peels and skins. It is acceptable to get an occasional serving of fruit in the form of juice. However, make sure that it is pure juice with no additional sugar added.

One serving of fruit is equal to ½ cup fresh cut-up fruit or berries, one medium-sized piece of fruit, or ½ cup of unsweetened fruit juice.

Dairy

Recommended servings: 2-3 per day

Dairy products like yogurt, milk, and cheese are excellent calcium and vitamin D, and protein sources. Yogurt and other dairy products that are gone through fermenting, such as kefir, also provide healthy gut bacteria to promote digestive health. Not only are strong bones and a healthy digestive system necessary, but research also conducted that puts vitamin D as a major player in protecting the body against certain cancers, not to mention its role in mental health. In some diets, dairy is seen as a taboo, high in fat, and irritating and inflammatory to the digestive system. Of course, if you have a lactose allergy or sensitivity, you should follow your guidelines for the inclusion or elimination of dairy in your daily diet. If your diet permits, lactose-free products are acceptable in the DASH Diet. One thing to keep in mind is that the dairy you choose should be low fat or fat-free. Full-fat dairy is calorie-dense and typically higher in sodium, but much of the fat you would consume is the saturated, unhealthy variety.

The one serving of dairy products should be 1 cup milk, 1 cup yogurt, 1 cup frozen yogurt, or 1 ½ ounce of cheese.

Lean Meats, Fish and Poultry

Recommended servings: 2 or less per day

You can't beat lean meats as a source of protein, iron, and B vitamins. However, even the leanest cuts of meats can be calorie-dense and high in fats and cholesterol. It is appropriate to include lean meats, fish, and poultry in your daily diet. However, they should not be the primary focus of each meal, as many of us in the Western world tend to do. The best way to incorporate these lean sources of protein is to begin by making them more of an accessory to your meals, rather than the star. Lesen the amount of meat and increase the number of fresh vegetables and grains. Trim away excess fat from meat and poultry and avoid cooking methods that require too much additional fat, such as frying.

The one serving of poultry, meat, or fish is equal to 3 ounces of fleshy meat or large poultry egg.

Nuts, Seeds, Legumes

Recommended servings: 4-5 per week

Nuts, which sometimes have a bad reputation due to their high calorie-per-serving ratio, are a heart-healthy addition to the diet. Nuts, seeds, and legumes all contain adequate amounts of fiber, protein, potassium, and magnesium, along with good omega-three fatty acids. Because these foods are plant-based, they contain phytochemicals, which are thought to help protect the body against cardiovascular disease and certain cancers. The trick to properly incorporating these foods into your diet is to keep portion size in mind. Nuts are delicious, and it can be easy to eat several handfuls without much thought. The problem with this is that those several handfuls add up to about three full servings and hundreds of calories. Choose nuts and seeds that are raw and unsalted for maximum health benefits.

A serving of nuts, seeds, or legumes is equal to 1 ½ ounce of nuts, ½ cup cooked beans, or approximately two tablespoons of seeds.

Fats and Oils

Recommended servings: 2-3 per day

It is essential to know that fat is not the enemy in the body — it helps protect our immune system, aids in the absorption of specific vitamins, and the right types of fat help protect the cardiovascular system. The problem with fat is a combination of the amount and kind found in the typical western diet. It is essential to focus on healthier unsaturated fats rather than saturated fats and trans fats, which are at least partly responsible for the ever-increasing heart disease and obesity epidemics. DASH guidelines suggest that no more than 25-27% of your daily caloric intake comes from fats and that those should be healthy (unsaturated) variety. Saturated fats should compose no more than 5-6% of your daily calories, so take it easy on full-fat dairy products.

One serving of fats and oils is equal to 1 teaspoon of oil, one tablespoon of mayonnaise, or two tablespoons of prepared salad dressing.

Sweet Treats

Recommended servings: 5 or less per week

The DASH Diet is not about giving up pleasures such as sweets and desserts, but rather rethinking your approach to them. There is nothing wrong with allowing a little sweetness in your life as long as you do not overindulge, and be mindful of your choices. Keep fruit as a centerpiece of your desserts, and when going decadent, choose rich, heart-healthy, dark chocolate. Foods such as high percentage cocoa chocolate, fruit sorbets and ices, hard candies, and fresh fruits will help to satisfy the sweet tooth without compromising your diet. Artificial sweeteners are acceptable, as long as you keep in mind that just because it isn't real sugar doesn't mean that you should overeat or replace more nutritious foods with artificially sweetened, less nutritional choices. Also, natural sugars are always best, so keep the artificially sweetened goods for special occasions and satisfy your cravings with a piece of poached fruit or a few squares of dark chocolate.

One serving of sweets is equal to ½ cup sorbet or fruit ice, one tablespoon jelly or jam, 1 cup sweetened fruit drink (such as limeade or lemonade), and ten candies as jelly beans, or 1 ½ ounce dark chocolate.

Chapter 21: Tips To Keep Blood Pressure Under Control; Reduce The Consumption Of Salt In The Kitchen To Stay Healthy.

Salt is so abundant in our diet, from bread to soups to sauces. Sodium is an essential mineral that performs many vital functions in your body. Sodium, the main component of salt, is a crucial nutrient. Increased sodium increases the risk of high blood pressure, leading to a heart attack or stroke.

It's usually found in foods such as eggs and vegetables, and table salt (sodium chloride) is also a key ingredient. While extremely important to health, for certain conditions, dietary sodium can sometimes be limited. For instance, a low-sodium diet is usually prescribed for people with certain medical conditions, including heart disease, hypertension, and kidney problems.

What Is A Low Sodium Diet?

Sodium involves in many vital functions of the human body, such as cellular functions, fluid regulation, electrolytes, and blood pressure maintenance. As this mineral is essential for life, the concentration (osmolarity) of body fluids is regulated precisely by your kidneys.

Across most of the food you eat, sodium is identified. Whole foods like vegetables, fruits, and chicken consist less. By contrast, foods based on plants, such as fresh food, usually have little sodium, unlike foods based on animals, such as dairy and meat products.

In processed food products such as French fries, frozen foods, and fast foods, sodium is most concentrated, while also salt is added throughout the process to enhance the flavor.

Adding salt to food when preparing a meal in your kitchen and seasoning it before eating is another crucial sodium intake factor. A low-sodium diet limits the foods and drinks which are high in sodium.

With a low-sodium diet, foods rich in sodium must be restricted or avoided entirely to keep the recommended sodium intake below the recommended level.

Tips for reducing your sodium intake

You ought to make a concerted effort not to include too many table salt when you go on a low-sodium diet. The food labels may require you to pay closer attention. High sodium foods are considered foods containing at least 20 percent of the recommended daily sodium allowance.

It is perceived that foods with no more than 5% of the recommended daily intake are low in sodium. There are a few simple additional options that can help in your diet to cut out sodium, in addition to reading food labels. Here are some simple tips for reducing your sodium intake:

- Look for low-sodium foods containing less than 120 mg of nutritional sodium.

- Instead of processed foods and snacks, choose fresh fruits and vegetables-fresh products are naturally low in sodium.

- Try to cook more often-processed foods are often loaded with sodium, frozen foods, and fast foods. Season your favorite meals with fresh herbs and dried spices to add flavor instead of salt.

- Pay more extra attention to the spices you mustard, use-ketchup, and salad dressings that usually comprise of high levels of sodium.

- When purchasing canned food, see for products that are labeled as 'low in sodium' or no salt added

- When cooking pasta, rice, or beans, do not apply salt in water and wash the canned beans before processing them.

Chapter 22: Menus to Rebalance Blood Pressure Values

Days	Breakfast	Luch	Dinner	Snack/Dessert
1	90 grams (1 cup) of oatmeal with 240 ml (1 cup) skim milk, 75 grams (1/2 cup) blueberries, 240 ml (1/2) orange juice (fresh)	Mayonnaise sandwich and tuna made with whole-grain bread (2 slices) mayonnaise, 15 grams (1 teaspoon), green salad, ½ cup (113 grams) and canned tuna, 80 grams (3 ounces)	Lean chicken breast, 85 grams (3 ounces) cooked in 5 ml (1 teaspoon) of vegetable oil with carrot and broccoli 75 grams (1/2 cup). And served with 1 cup of brown rice (190 grams)	Apple: 1 medium and 250 grams (1 cup) of low-fat sugar. Banana:1 medium

2	Whole-wheat toast, two slices with 4.5 grams of margarine (1 teaspoon), jam or jelly, one teaspoon (20 grams), one apple (medium), fresh orange juice, ½ cup (120 ml)	Lean chicken breast, 85 grams (3 ounces) with a green salad, 150 grams (2 cups), low-fat cheese, 45 grams (1.5 ounces), and one cup of brown rice (150 grams)	85 grams of salmon (3 ounces) cooked vegetable oil, ml (1 teaspoon) with boiled potatoes, 300 grams (1 cup) and boiled vegetables, 225 grams (1.5 cups)	Canned peaches, 30 grams (1/2 cup) and low-fat yogurt, 285 grams (1 cup) Banana: 1 medium	
3	90 grams (1 cup) of oatmeal with skim milk, 1 cup (240 ml)) and blueberries, ½ cup (75 grams) and orange juice, ½	Whole wheat bread, two slices. Lean Turkey, 85 grams (3 ounces). Low fat cheese, 45 grams (1.5 ounces),	Cod fillets, 170 grams (6 ounces) with mashed potatoes, 200 grams (1 cup) green peas, 76	Orange: 1 medium Whole-grain crackers, 1 with cottage cheese, 45 grams (1.5 ounces) and canned pineapple, 75	

	cup (120 ml)	green salad, 38 grams (1/2 cup) and cherry tomatoes, 38 grams (1/2 cup)	grams (1/2 cup) and broccoli, 75 grams (1/2 cup)	grams (1/2 cup)
4	Oatmeal, 90 grams (1 cup) with skim milk, 240 ml (1 cup) and raspberries, 75 grams (1/2 cup) and fresh orange juice, 120 ml (1/2 cup)	Salad prepared with 130 grams (4.5 ounces) of grilled tuna, boiled egg 1, green salad, 152 grams (2 cups), cherry tomatoes, 38 grams (1/2 cup) and low-fat dressing, 30 ml (2 tablespoons)	Pork fillets, 85 grams (3 ounces) with mixed vegetables, 150 grams (1 cup) and brown rice, 190 grams, (1 cup)	Banana: 1 medium Can pears, 30 grams (1/2) and low-fat yogurt 285 grams (1 cup)
5	Boiled eggs 2, turkey bacon, two	Whole wheat toast two	Spaghetti and meatballs	Apple: 1, medium

	slices, cherry tomatoes, 38 grams (1/2 cup) baked beans, 80 grams (1/2 cup) whole-wheat toast, two pieces, and orange juice, 120ml, (1/2 cup)	slices, low-fat mayonnaise, one tablespoon, low-fat cheese, 45 grams (1.5 ounces), salad greens, 38 grams (1/2 cup) and cherry tomatoes, 38 grams (1/2 cup)	prepared with spaghetti, 190 grams (1 cup), and minced turkey 115 grams (4 ounces) with 75 grams (1/2 cup) green beans on the side.	Fruit salad: 1 cup
6	Whole wheat toast, two slices, with peanut butter, 40 grams (2 tablespoons), banana, one medium, mixed seeds, 16 grams (2 tablespoons) and	Grilled chicken, 85 grams (3 ounces), roasted vegetables 150 grams (1 cup) and couscous 190 grams (1 cup)	Pork steak 85 grams ((3 ounces) and ratatouille 150 gram (1 cup) with brown rice 190 grams (1 cup), lentils 40 grams (1/2 cup),	Apple: 1, medium Mixed berries, 30 grams (1/2 cup) and low-fat yogurt, 285 grams (1 cup) Chocolate pudding low-fat.

	orange juice, 120 ml (1/2 cup)		and low-fat cheese 45grams (1/2 cup)	
7	Oatmeal 90 grams (1 cup) with skim milk 240 ml (1 cup), blueberries 75 grams (1/2 cup), orange juice 240 ml (1/2 cup)	Chicken salad prepared with 85 grams (3 ounces) of lean chicken breast, mayonnaise one tablespoon, green salad 150 g grams (2 cups), cherry tomatoes 75 grams (1/2 cup), seeds 4 grams (1/2 tablespoon), and whole-grain crackers 4.	Roast beef 3 ounces with boiled potatoes 150 grams (1 cup), broccoli 75 grams (1)2 cup) and green peas 75g (1/2 cup)	Pear: 1 medium Banana 1 and almond 70 grams (1/2 cup)

| 8 | Whole wheat bagel: 1, (store-bought) with peanut butter two tablespoons (no salt) Orange: 1 medium Fat-free milk: 1 cup Coffee, decaffeinated. | Spinach salad prepared with Spinach leaves, fresh: 4; cups Sliced pear: 1 Canned Mandarin ½ cup Almond, silvered: 1/3 cup Red wine vinaigrette : 2 tablespoons | Baked cod, herb-crusted: 4 ounces raw (about 3 ounces cooked) Vegetables with brown rice pilaf: ½ cup Steamed, fresh green beans: ½ cup Sourdough roll: 1, small Olive oil: 2 teaspoons Chopped mint with fresh Berry. 1 cup | Wheat crackers: 12, sodium-reduced. Fat-free milk: 1 cup Low-calorie yogurt, fat-free: 1 cup. Vanilla wafers: 4 |

			Ice tea, herbal.	
9	Fresh mixed fruits like banana, apple, melon, and berries 1 cup with low calorie, fat-free vanilla yogurt 1 cup, and walnuts 1/3 cup Bran muffin: 1 Trans-free margarine: 1 teaspoon. Fat-free milk: 1 cup Herbal tea.	Curried chicken wrap prepared with: Whole wheat tortilla: 1 medium Three ounces of chopped chicken. Chopped apple: ½ cup Light mayonnaise: 1 ½ Tablespoon curry powder: 1/2 teaspoon Snack	Whole wheat spaghetti, 1 cup with marinara sauce, 1 cup (no salt) Salad greens, mixed: 2 cups Low-fat Caesar Dressing: 1 tablespoon Whole-wheat roll: 1 small Olive oil: 1 teaspoon Nectarine: 1	Trial mix prepared with Raisins: ¼ cup Mini twist pretzels, unsalted, 1 ounce (about 22) Sunflower seeds: 2 tablespoons

		8 baby berries, raw: 1/2 cup Fat-free milk: 1 cup	Sparkling water.	
10	Cooked oatmeal, old fashioned: 1 cup with topped with cinnamon 1 one teaspoon Whole wheat toast, sliced: 1 Trans free margarine: 1 teaspoon Banana: 1 Fat-free milk: 1 cup	Tuna prepared with water-packed tuna, drained, ½ cup (unsalted) Light mayonnaise: 2 tablespoons Grapes: 15 Celery, diced: ¼ cup Sat on top of romaine lettuce: 2 ½ cups	Vegetable kebab and beef, prepared with: Beef: 3 ounces Cherry tomatoes, onions, peppers, and mushrooms: 1 cup Wild rice, cooked: 1 cup. Pecans: 1/3 cup Pineapple chunks: 1 cup	Melba toast crackers: 8 Fat-free milk: 1 cup Light yogurt: 1 cup. Peach: 1, medium

		Snack Melba toast crackers: 8 Fat-free milk: 1 cup	Cran raspberry spritzer prepared with Cran-raspberry juice: 4 ounces Sparkling water: 4-8 ounces	
11	Whole-wheat toast, two slices with 4.5 grams of margarine (1 teaspoon), jam or jelly, one teaspoon (20 grams), one apple (medium), fresh orange juice, ½	Lean chicken breast, 85 grams (3 ounces) with a green salad, 150 grams (2 cups), low-fat cheese, 45 grams (1.5 ounces), and one cup of brown rice	85 grams of salmon (3 ounces) cooked vegetable oil, ml (1 teaspoon) with boiled potatoes, 300 grams (1 cup) and boiled vegetables, 225	Banana: 1 medium Canned peaches, 30 grams (1/2 cup) and low-fat yogurt, 285 grams (1 cup)

	cup (120 ml)	(150 grams)	grams (1.5 cups)	
12	90 grams (1 cup) of oatmeal with skim milk, 1 cup (240 ml)) and blueberries, ½ cup (75 grams) and orange juice, ½ cup (120 ml)	Whole wheat bread, two slices. Lean Turkey, 85 grams (3 ounces). Low-fat cheese, 45 grams (1.5 ounces), green salad, 38 grams (1/2 cup) and cherry tomatoes, 38 grams (1/2 cup)	Cod fillets, 170 grams (6 ounces) with mashed potatoes, 200 grams (1 cup) green peas, 76 grams (1/2 cup) and broccoli, 75 grams (1/2 cup, medium)	Orange: 1 medium Whole-grain crackers, 4 with cottage cheese, 45 grams (1.5 ounces) and canned pineapple, 75 grams (1/2 cup)

Chapter 23: Anti-Hypertension Appetizers Recipes

Carrot, Ginger, and Turmeric Soup

Preparation Time: 15 minutes

Cooking Time: 40 minutes

Serving: 4

Ingredients:

6 cups chicken broth

¼ cup full-fat coconut milk, unsweetened

¾ pound carrots, peeled and chopped

One teaspoon turmeric, ground

Two teaspoons ginger, grated

One yellow onion, chopped

Two garlic cloves, peeled

Pinch of pepper

Directions:

Take a stockpot and add all the ingredients except coconut milk into it.

Place stockpot over medium heat.

Bring to a boil.

Reduce heat to simmer for 40 minutes.

Remove the bay leaf.

Blend the soup until smooth by using an immersion blender.

Add the coconut milk and stir.

Serve immediately and enjoy!

Nutrition:

Calories: 79

Fat: 4g

Carbohydrates: 7g

Protein: 4g

Offbeat Squash Soup

Preparation Time: 10 minutes

Cooking Time: 50 minutes

Serving: 4

Ingredients:

One butternut squash, cut in half lengthwise and deseeded

14 ounces of coconut milk

Pinch of salt

Black pepper to taste

A handful of parsley, chopped

Pinch of nutmeg, ground

Directions

Add butternut squash halves on a lined baking sheet.

Place in oven and bake for 45 minutes at 350 degrees F.

Leave squash to cool down and scoop out the flesh to a pot.

Add half of the coconut milk to the pot and blend using an immersion blender.

Heat soup over medium-low heat and add remaining coconut milk.

Add a pinch of salt, black pepper to taste.

Add nutmeg, parsley, and blend using an immersion blender once again for a few seconds.

Cook for 4 minutes.

Serve and enjoy!

Nutrition:

Calories: 144

Fat: 10g

Carbohydrates: 7g

Protein: 2g

Leek and Cauliflower Soup

Preparation Time: 10 minutes

Cooking Time: 40 minutes

Serving: 6

Ingredients:

3 cups cauliflower, riced

One bay leaf

One teaspoon herbs de Provence

Two garlic cloves, peeled and diced

½ cup of coconut milk

2 ½ cups vegetable stock

One tablespoon coconut oil

½ teaspoon cracked pepper

One leek, chopped

Directions:

Take a pot, heat oil into it.

Sauté the leeks in the oil for 5 minutes.

Add the garlic, and then stir-cook for another minute.

Add all the remaining ingredients and mix them well.

Cook for 30 minutes.

Stir occasionally.

Blend the soup until smooth by using an immersion blender.

Serve hot and enjoy!

Nutrition:

Calories: 90

Fat: 7g

Carbohydrates: 4g

Protein: 2g

Dreamy Zucchini Bowl

Preparation Time: 10 minutes

Cooking Time: 20 minutes

Serving: 4

Ingredients:

One onion, chopped

Three zucchini, cut into medium chunks

Two tablespoons coconut almond milk

Two garlic cloves, minced

4 cups vegetable stock

Two tablespoons coconut oil

Pinch of sunflower seeds

Black pepper to taste

Direction:

Take a pot and place it over medium heat.

Add oil and let it heat up.

Add zucchini, garlic, onion, and stir.

Cook for 5 minutes.

Add stock, sunflower seeds, pepper, and stir.

Bring to a boil and reduce heat.

Simmer for 20 minutes.

Remove from heat and add coconut almond milk.

Use an immersion blender until smooth.

Ladle into soup bowls and serve.

Enjoy!

Nutrition:

Calories: 160

Fat: 2g

Carbohydrates: 4g

Protein: 7g

Cold Crab and Watermelon Soup

Preparation Time: 10 minutes + chill time

Cooking Time: 0 minutes

Serving: 4

Ingredients:

¼ cup basil, chopped

2 pounds tomatoes

5 cups watermelon, cubed

¼ cup wine vinegar

Two garlic cloves, minced

One zucchini, chopped

Pepper to taste

1 cup crabmeat

Direction

Take your blender and add tomatoes, basil, vinegar, 4 cups watermelon, garlic, 1/3 cup oil, pepper, and pulse well.

Put it in the fridge and chill for 1 hour.

Divide into bowls and add zucchini, crab, and remaining watermelon.

Serve and enjoy!

Nutrition:

Calories: 121

Fat: 3g

Carbohydrates: 4g

Protein: 8g

Paleo Lemon and Garlic Soup

Preparation Time: 10 minutes

Cooking Time: 10 minutes

Serving: 4

Ingredients:

6 cups shellfish stock

One tablespoon garlic, minced

One tablespoon coconut oil, melted

Two whole eggs

½ cup lemon juice

Pinch of salt

White pepper to taste

One tablespoon arrowroot powder

Finely chopped cilantro for serving

Directions:

Heat a pot with oil over medium-high heat.

Add garlic, stir cook for 2 minutes.

Add stock (reserve ½ cup for later use).

Stir and bring the mix to a simmer.

Take a bowl and add eggs, sea salt, pepper, reserved stock, lemon juice, and arrowroot.

Whisk well.

Pour into the soup and cook for a few minutes.

Ladle soup into bowls and serve with chopped cilantro.

Enjoy!

Nutrition:

Calories: 135

Fat: 3g

Carbohydrates: 12g

Protein: 8

Brussels Soup

Preparation Time: 10 minutes

Cooking Time: 20 minutes

Serving: 4

Ingredients:

Two tablespoons olive oil

One yellow onion, chopped

2 pounds Brussels sprouts, trimmed and halved

4 cups chicken stock

¼ cup coconut cream

Directions:

Take a pot and place it over medium heat.

Add oil and let it heat up.

Add onion and stir cook for 3 minutes.

Add Brussels sprouts and stir, cook for 2 minutes.

Add stock and black pepper, stir and bring to a simmer.

Cook for 20 minutes more.

Use an immersion blender to make the soup creamy.

Add coconut cream and stir well.

Ladle into soup bowls and serve.

Enjoy!

Nutrition:

Calories: 200

Fat: 11g

Carbohydrates: 6g

Protein: 11g

Spring Soup and Poached Egg

Preparation Time: 5 minutes

Cooking Time: 15 minutes

Serving: 4

Ingredients:

Two whole eggs

32 ounces chicken broth

One head romaine lettuce, chopped

Directions:

Bring the chicken broth to a boil.

Reduce the heat and poach the two eggs in the broth for 5 minutes.

Take two bowls and transfer the eggs into a separate bowl.

Add chopped romaine lettuce into the broth and cook for a few minutes.

Serve the broth with lettuce into the bowls.

Enjoy!

Nutrition:

Calories: 150

Fat: 5g

Carbohydrates: 6g

Protein: 16g

Lobster Bisque

Preparation Time: 10 minutes

Cooking Time: 15 minutes

Serving: 4

Ingredients:

¾ pound lobster, cooked and lobster

4 cups chicken broth

Two garlic cloves, chopped

¼ teaspoon pepper

½ teaspoon paprika

One yellow onion, chopped

½ teaspoon salt

14 ½ ounces tomatoes, diced

One tablespoon coconut oil

1 cup low fat cream

Directions:

Take a stockpot and add the coconut oil over medium heat.

Then sauté the garlic and onion for 3 to 5 minutes.

Add diced tomatoes, spices, and chicken broth and bring to a boil.

Reduce to a simmer, then simmer for about 10 minutes.

Add the warmed heavy cream to the soup.

Blend the soup till creamy by using an immersion blender.

Stir in cooked lobster.

Serve and enjoy!

Nutrition:

Calories: 180

Fat: 11g

Carbohydrates: 6g

Protein: 16g

Tomato Bisque

Preparation Time: 10 minutes

Cooking Time: 40 minutes

Serving: 4

Ingredients:

4 cups chicken broth

1 cup low fat cream

One teaspoon thyme dried

3 cups canned whole, peeled tomatoes

Two tablespoons almond butter

Three garlic cloves, peeled

Pepper as needed

Directions:

Take a stockpot and first add the butter to the bottom of a stockpot.

Then add all the ingredients except heavy cream into it.

Bring to a boil.

Simmer for 40 minutes.

Warm the heavy cream and stir into the soup.

Serve and enjoy!

Nutrition:

Calories: 141

Fat: 12g

Carbohydrates: 4g

Protein: 4g

Chipotle Chicken Chowder

Preparation Time: 10 minutes

Cooking Time: 23 minutes

Serving: 4

Ingredients:

One medium onion, chopped

Two garlic cloves, minced

Six bacon slices, chopped

4 cups jicama, cubed

3 cups chicken stock

One teaspoon salt

2 cups low-fat cream

One tablespoon olive oil

Two tablespoons fresh cilantro, chopped

One ¼ pounds chicken, thigh boneless, cut into 1-inch chunks

½ teaspoon pepper

One chipotle pepper, minced

Directions:

Heat the olive oil in medium heat large-sized saucepan, add bacon.

Cook until crispy, add onion, garlic, and jicama.

Cook for 7 minutes, add chicken stock and chicken.

Bring to a boil and reduce temperature to low.

Simmer for 10 minutes

Season with salt and pepper.

Add heavy cream and chipotle, simmer for 5 minutes.

Sprinkle chopped cilantro and serve, enjoy!

Nutrition:

Calories: 350

Fat: 22g

Carbohydrates: 8g

Protein: 22g

Bay Scallop Chowder

Preparation Time: 10 minutes

Cooking Time: 18 minutes

Serving: 4

Ingredients:

One medium onion, chopped

2 ½ cups chicken stock

Four slices bacon, chopped

3 cups daikon radish, chopped

½ teaspoon dried thyme

2 cups low-fat cream

One tablespoon almond butter

Pepper to taste

1 pound bay scallops

Directions:

Heat olive over medium heat in a large-sized saucepan, add bacon and cook until crisp, add onion and daikon radish.

Cook for 5 minutes, add chicken stock.

Simmer for 8 minutes, season with salt and pepper, thyme.

Add heavy cream, bay scallops, simmer for 4 minutes

Serve and enjoy!

Nutrition:

Calories: 307

Fat: 22g

Carbohydrates: 7g

Protein: 22g

Salmon and Vegetable Soup

Preparation Time: 10 minutes

Cooking Time: 22 minutes

Serving: 4

Ingredients:

Two tablespoons extra-virgin olive oil

One leek, chopped

One red onion, chopped

Pepper to taste

Two carrots, chopped

4 cups low stock vegetable stock

4 ounces salmon, skinless and boneless, cubed

½ cup coconut cream

One tablespoon dill, chopped

Directions:

Place the pan over medium heat, add leek, onion, stir and cook for 7 minutes.

Add pepper, carrots, stock, and stir.

Boil for 10 minutes.

Add salmon, cream, dill, and stir.

Boil for 5-6 minutes.

Ladle into bowls and serve.

Enjoy!

Nutrition:

Calories: 240

Fat: 4g

Carbohydrates: 7g

Protein: 12g

Garlic Tomato Soup

Preparation Time: 15 minutes

Cooking Time: 15 minutes

Serving: 4

Ingredients:

8 Roma tomatoes, chopped

1 cup tomatoes, sundried

Two tablespoons coconut oil

Five garlic cloves, chopped

14 ounces of coconut milk

1 cup vegetable broth

Pepper to taste

Basil, for garnish

Directions:

Take a pot, heat oil into it.

Sauté the garlic in it for ½ minute.

Mix in the Roma tomatoes and cook for 8-10 minutes.

Stir occasionally.

Except for the basil, add the rest of the ingredients and stir well.

Cover the lid and cook for 5 minutes.

Let it cool.

Blend the soup until smooth by using an immersion blender.

Garnish with basil. Serve and enjoy!

Nutrition:

Calories: 240

Fat: 23g

Carbohydrates: 16g

Protein: 7g

Melon Soup

Preparation Time: 6 minutes

Cooking Time: 0 minutes

Serving: 4

Ingredients:

4 cups casaba melon, seeded and cubed

One tablespoon fresh ginger, grated

¾ cup of coconut milk

Juice of 2 limes

Direction:

Add the lime juice, coconut milk, casaba melon, ginger, and salt into your blender.

Blend it for 1-2 minutes or until you get a smooth mixture.

Serve and enjoy!

Nutrition:

Calories: 134

Fat: 9g

Carbohydrates: 13g

Protein: 2g

Chapter 24: Anti-Hypertension First Course Recipes

Pistachio Quinoa Salad with Pomegranate Citrus Vinaigrette

Preparation Time: 15 minutes

Cooking time: 15 minutes

Servings: 6

Ingredients

The Quinoa

1½ cups water

1 cup quinoa

¼ teaspoon kosher salt

For The Dressing

1 cup extra-virgin olive oil

½ cup pomegranate juice

½ cup freshly squeezed orange juice

One small shallot, minced

One teaspoon pure maple syrup

One teaspoon za'atar

½ teaspoon ground sumac

½ teaspoon kosher salt

¼ teaspoon freshly ground black pepper

The Salad

3 cups baby spinach

½ cup fresh parsley, coarsely chopped

½ cup fresh mint, coarsely chopped

Approximately ¾ cup pomegranate seeds, or two pomegranates

¼ cup pistachios shelled and toasted

¼ cup crumbled blue cheese

Direction:

Bring the water, quinoa, and salt to a boil in a small saucepan. Reduce the heat and cover; simmer for 10 to 12 minutes. Fluff with a fork.

To Make The Dressing:

In a medium bowl, whisk together the olive oil, pomegranate juice, orange juice, shallot, maple syrup, za'atar, sumac, salt, and black pepper. In a large bowl, add about ½ cup of dressing.

Store the remaining dressing in a glass jar or airtight container and refrigerate. The sauce can be kept up to 2 weeks.

Let the chilled dressing reach room temperature before using it.

To Make The Salad:

Combine the spinach, parsley, and mint in the bowl with the dressing and toss gently together. Add the quinoa. Toss gently. Add the pomegranate seeds.

Or, if using whole pomegranates: Cut the pomegranates in half. Fill a large bowl with water and hold the pomegranate half, cut-side-down.

Using a wooden spoon, hit the pomegranate's back, so the seeds fall into the water. Immerse the pomegranate in the water and gently pull out any remaining seeds.

Repeat with the remaining pomegranate. Skim the white pith off the top of the water. Rinse the seeds and add them to the greens. Add the pistachios and cheese and toss gently.

Nutrition:

Calories: 300

Total fat: 19g

Saturated fat: 4g

Cholesterol: 6mg

Total Carbohydrates: 28g

Cauliflower Tabbouleh Salad

Preparation Time: 15 minutes

Cooking time: 0 minutes

Servings: 4

Ingredients

¼ cup extra-virgin olive oil

¼ cup lemon juice

Zest of 1 lemon

¾ teaspoon kosher salt

½ teaspoon ground turmeric

¼ teaspoon ground coriander

¼ teaspoon ground cumin

¼ teaspoon black pepper

⅛ teaspoon ground cinnamon

1 pound riced cauliflower

1 English cucumber, diced

12 cherry tomatoes, halved

1 cup fresh parsley, chopped

½ cup fresh mint, chopped

Directions:

Whisk together the olive oil, lemon juice, lemon zest, salt, turmeric, coriander, cumin, black pepper, and cinnamon in a large bowl. Add the riced cauliflower to the bowl and mix well. Add in the cucumber, tomatoes, parsley, and mint and gently mix.

Nutrition:

Calories: 180

Total fat: 15g

Total Carbohydrates

Protein: 4g

Tuna Niçoise

Preparation Time: 15 minutes

Cooking time: 20 minutes

Servings: 4

Ingredients

1 pound small red or fingerling potatoes, halved

1 pound green beans or haricots verts, trimmed

One head romaine lettuce, chopped or torn into bite-size pieces

½ pint cherry tomatoes halved

Eight radishes, sliced thin

½ cup olives, pitted (any kind you like)

2 (5-ounce) cans no-salt-added tuna packed in olive oil, drained

Eight anchovies (optional)

Directions:

With a steamer basket with 2 to 3 inches of water, fill a large pot. Put the potatoes in the steamer basket and lay the green beans on top of the potatoes.

Wait for the water to a boil over high heat, lower the heat to low and simmer, cover, and cook for 7 minutes, or until the green beans are tender but crisp.

Remove the green beans and continue to steam the potatoes for an additional 10 minutes.

Place the romaine lettuce on a serving platter. Group the potatoes, green beans, tomatoes, radishes, olives, and tuna in different areas of the platter

Nutrition:

Calories: 315

Total fat: 9g

Total Carbohydrates: 33g

Protein: 28g

Roasted Golden Beet, Avocado, and Watercress Salad

Preparation Time: 15 minutes

Cooking time: 1 hour

Servings: 4

Ingredients

One bunch (about 1½ pounds) golden beets

One tablespoon extra-virgin olive oil

One tablespoon white wine vinegar

½ teaspoon kosher salt

¼ teaspoon freshly ground black pepper

One bunch (about 4 ounces) watercress

One avocado, peeled, pitted, and diced

¼ cup crumbled feta cheese

¼ cup walnuts, toasted

One tablespoon fresh chives, chopped

Directions:

Preheat the oven to 425°F. Wash and trim the beets (cut an inch above the beetroot, leaving the long tail if desired), then wrap each beet individually in foil.

In a baking sheet, put the beets and roast until fully cooked, 45 to 60 minutes depending on each beet's size. Start checking at 45 minutes; if easily pierced with a fork, the beets are cooked.

Remove the beets from the oven and allow them to cool. Under cold running water, slough off the skin. Cut the beets into bite-size cubes or wedges.

Whisk together the olive oil, vinegar, salt, and black pepper in a large bowl. Add the watercress and beets and toss well. Add the avocado, feta, walnuts, and chives and mix gently.

Nutrition:

Calories: 235

Total fat: 16g

Protein: 6g

Wild Rice Salad with Chickpeas and Pickled Radish

Preparation Time: 20 minutes

Cooking time: 45 minutes

Servings: 4-6

Ingredients

For The Rice

1 cup of water

4 ounces (⅔ cup) wild rice

¼ teaspoon kosher salt

For The Pickled Radish

One bunch radishes (6 to 8 small), sliced thin

½ cup white wine vinegar

½ teaspoon kosher salt

For The Dressing

Two tablespoons extra-virgin olive oil

Two tablespoons white wine vinegar

½ teaspoon pure maple syrup

½ teaspoon kosher salt

¼ teaspoon freshly ground black pepper

The Salad

1 (15-ounce) can no-salt-added or low-sodium chickpeas, rinsed and drained

One bulb fennel, diced

¼ cup walnuts, chopped and toasted

¼ cup crumbled feta cheese

¼ cup currants

Two tablespoons fresh dill, chopped

To Make The Rice

Bring the water, rice, and salt to a boil in a medium saucepan. Cover, reduce the heat and simmer for 45 minutes.

To Make The Pickled Radish

In a medium bowl, combine the radishes, vinegar, and salt. Let sit for 15 to 30 minutes.

To Make The Dressing

Whisk together the olive oil, vinegar, maple syrup, salt, and black pepper in a large bowl.

To Make The Salad

While still warm, add the rice to the bowl with the dressing and mix well. Add the chickpeas, fennel, walnuts, feta, currants, and dill. Mix well. Garnish with the pickled radishes before serving.

Nutrition:

Calories: 310

Total fat: 16g

Total Carbohydrates: 36g

Protein: 10g

Quinoa with Zucchini, Mint, and Pistachios

Preparation Time: 20-30 minutes

Cooking time: 20 minutes

Servings: 4

Ingredients

The Quinoa

1½ cups water

1 cup quinoa

¼ teaspoon kosher salt

The Salad

Two tablespoons extra-virgin olive oil

One zucchini, thinly sliced into rounds

Six small radishes, sliced

One shallot, julienned

¾ teaspoon kosher salt

¼ teaspoon freshly ground black pepper

Two garlic cloves, sliced

Zest of 1 lemon

Two tablespoons lemon juice

¼ cup fresh mint, chopped

¼ cup fresh basil, chopped

¼ cup pistachios shelled and toasted

Directions:

In a medium saucepan, bring the water, quinoa, and salt to a boil. Reduce to a simmer, cover, and cook for 10 to 12 minutes. Fluff with a fork.

Heat the olive oil in a large skillet or sauté pan over medium-high heat. Add the zucchini, radishes, shallot, salt, black pepper, and sauté for 7 to 8 minutes.

Then, add the garlic and cook 30 seconds to 1 minute more.

In a large bowl, combine the lemon zest and lemon juice. Add the quinoa and mix well. Add the cooked zucchini mixture and mix well. Add the mint, basil, and pistachios and gently mix.

Nutrition:
Calories: 220
Total fat: 12g
Total Carbohydrates: 25g
Protein: 6g

Italian White Bean Salad with Bell Peppers

Preparation Time: 15 minutes

Cooking time: 0 minutes

Servings: 4

Ingredients

Two tablespoons extra-virgin olive oil

Two tablespoons white wine vinegar

½ shallot, minced

½ teaspoon kosher salt

¼ teaspoon freshly ground black pepper

3 cups of cooked cannellini beans or two cans no-salt-added or low-sodium cannellini beans, drained and rinsed

Two celery stalks, diced

½ red bell pepper, diced

¼ cup fresh parsley, chopped

¼ cup fresh mint, chopped

Directions:

Whisk together the olive oil, vinegar, shallot, salt, and black pepper in a large bowl. Add the beans, celery, red bell pepper, parsley, and mint; mix well.

Nutrition:

Calories: 300;

Total fat: 8g;

Total Carbohydrates: 46g;

Protein: 15g;

French Lentil Salad with Parsley and Mint

Preparation Time: 20 minutes

Cooking time: 25 minutes

Servings: 4-6

Ingredients

For The Lentils

1 cup French lentils

One garlic clove smashed

One dried bay leaf

The Salad

Two tablespoons extra-virgin olive oil

Two tablespoons red wine vinegar

½ teaspoon ground cumin

½ teaspoon kosher salt

¼ teaspoon freshly ground black pepper

Two celery stalks, diced small

One bell pepper, diced small

½ red onion, diced small

¼ cup fresh parsley, chopped

¼ cup fresh mint, chopped

Directions:

To Make The Lentils

In a large saucepan, put the lentils, garlic, and bay leaf. Cover with water by about 3 inches and bring to a boil. Reduce the heat, cover, and simmer until tender, 20 to 30 minutes.

Drain the lentils to remove any remaining water after cooking. Remove the garlic and bay leaf.

To Make The Salad

Whisk together the olive oil, vinegar, cumin, salt, and black pepper in a large bowl. Add the celery, bell pepper, onion, parsley, and mint and toss to combine. Add the lentils and mix well.

Nutrition:

Calories: 200;

Total fat: 8g;

Saturated fat: 1g;

Total Carbohydrates: 26g;

Protein: 10g

Roasted Cauliflower and Arugula Salad with Pomegranate and Pine Nuts

Preparation Time: 20 minutes

Cooking time: 20 minutes

Servings: 4

Ingredients

One head cauliflower, trimmed and cut into 1-inch florets

Two tablespoons extra-virgin olive oil, plus more for drizzling (optional)

One teaspoon ground cumin

½ teaspoon kosher salt

¼ teaspoon freshly ground black pepper

5 ounces arugula

⅓ cup pomegranate seeds

¼ cup pine nuts, toasted

Directions:

Preheat the oven to 425°F. Line parchment paper or foil in a baking sheet. In a large bowl, combine the cauliflower, olive oil, cumin, salt, and black pepper. Spread in a single layer on the prepared baking sheet and roast for 20 minutes, tossing halfway through.

Divide the arugula among four plates. Top with the cauliflower, pomegranate seeds, and pine nuts. Serve with Lemon Vinaigrette dressing or a simple drizzle of olive oil.

Nutrition:

Calories: 190

Total fat: 14g

Total Carbohydrates: 16g

Protein: 6g;

Red Gazpacho

Preparation Time: 15 minutes

Cooking time: 0 minutes

Servings: 4

Ingredients

2 pounds tomatoes, cut into chunks

One bell pepper, cut into chunks

One cucumber, cut into chunks

One small red onion, cut into chunks

One garlic clove smashed

Two teaspoons sherry vinegar

½ teaspoon kosher salt

¼ teaspoon freshly ground black pepper

⅓ cup extra-virgin olive oil

Lemon juice (optional)

¼ cup fresh chives, chopped, for garnish

Directions:

Add the tomatoes, bell pepper, cucumber, onion, garlic, vinegar, salt, and black pepper in a high-speed blender or Vitamix.

Blend until smooth. With the motor running, add the olive oil and purée until smooth. Add more vinegar or a spritz of lemon juice if needed. Garnish with the chives.

Nutrition:

Calories: 240

Total fat: 19g

Total Carbohydrates: 18g

Protein: 4

Chapter 25: Anti- Hypertension Second Course Recipes

Moroccan-Inspired Tagine with Chickpeas & Vegetables

Preparation Time: 10 minutes

Cooking time: 45 minutes

Servings: 2-3

Ingredients

Two teaspoons olive oil

1 cup chopped carrots

½ cup finely chopped onion

One sweet potato, diced

1 cup low-sodium vegetable broth

¼ teaspoon ground cinnamon

⅛ teaspoon salt

1½ cups chopped bell peppers, any color

Three ripe plum tomatoes, seeded and finely chopped

One tablespoon tomato paste

One garlic clove, pressed or minced

1 (15-ounce) can chickpeas, drained and rinsed

½ cup chopped dried apricots

One teaspoon curry powder

½ teaspoon paprika

½ teaspoon turmeric

Directions:

Heat the oil over medium heat in a large Dutch oven or saucepan. Next, add the carrots and onion. Cook it until the onion is translucent about 4 minutes.

Add the sweet potato, broth, cinnamon, and salt and cook for 5 to 6 minutes, until the broth is slightly reduced.

Add the peppers, tomatoes, tomato paste, and garlic. Stir and cook for another 5 minutes. Add the chickpeas, apricots, curry powder, paprika, and turmeric to the pot.

Bring all to a boil, then reduce the heat to low, cover, simmer for about 30 minutes, and serve.

Nutrition:

Calories 469

Total Fat: 9g

Carbohydrates: 88g

Protein: 16g

Spaghetti Squash with Maple Glaze & Tofu Crumbles

Preparation Time: 20 minutes

Cooking time: 22 minutes

Servings: 2-3

Ingredients:

2 ounces firm tofu, well-drained

One small spaghetti squash halved lengthwise

2½ teaspoons olive oil, divided

⅛ teaspoon salt

½ cup chopped onion

One teaspoon dried rosemary

¼ cup dry white wine

Two tablespoons maple syrup

½ teaspoon garlic powder

¼ cup shredded Gruyère cheese

Directions:

Put the tofu in a large mesh colander and place over a large bowl to drain. Use a paring knife to score the squash so the steam can vent while it cooks.

Place the squash in a medium microwave-safe dish and microwave on high for 5 minutes. Remove the squash from the microwave and allow it to cool.

Cut the cooled squash in half on a cutting board. Scoop out the seeds, then place the squash halves into a 9-by-11-inch baking dish.

Drizzle the squash with half a teaspoon of olive oil, season it with the salt, then cover it with wax paper, put it back in the microwave for five more minutes on high, or until the skin is easily pierced with a fork.

Once it's cooked, scrape the squash strands with a fork into a small bowl and cover it to keep it warm. While the squash is cooking, heat one teaspoon of oil in a large skillet over medium-high heat. Add the onion and sauté for 5 minutes.

Add the rosemary and stir for 1 minute, until fragrant. In the same skillet, add the remaining oil. Crumble the tofu into the skillet, stir fry until lightly browned, about 4 minutes, and transfer it to a small bowl.

Add the wine, maple syrup, and garlic powder to the skillet and stir to combine. Cook for 2 minutes until slightly reduced and thickened. Remove from the heat.

Evenly divide the squash between two plates, then top it with the tofu mixture. Drizzle the maple glaze over the top, then add the grated cheese.

Nutrition:

Calories 330

Total fat: 15g

Carbohydrates: 36g

Protein: 12g

Stuffed Tex-Mex Baked Potatoes

Preparation Time: 10 minutes

Cooking time: 45 minutes

Servings: 2

Ingredients

Two large Idaho potatoes

½ cup black beans, rinsed and drained

¼ cup store-bought salsa

One avocado, diced

One teaspoon freshly squeezed lime juice

½ cup nonfat plain Greek yogurt

¼ teaspoon reduced-sodium taco seasoning

¼ cup shredded sharp cheddar cheese

Directions:

Preheat the oven to 400°F. Scrub the potatoes. Cut an "X" into the top of each using a paring knife. Place the potatoes directly on the oven rack and bake for 45 minutes until they are tender.

In a small bowl, stir together the beans and salsa and set aside. In another small bowl, mix the avocado and lime juice and set aside.

Stir together the yogurt and the taco seasoning until well blended in a third small bowl. When the potatoes are baked, carefully open them up.

Top each potato with the bean and salsa mixture, avocado, seasoned yogurt, and cheddar cheese, evenly dividing each component, and serve.

Nutrition:

Calories 624

Total fat: 21g

Carbohydrates: 91g

Fiber: 21g

Protein: 24g

Lentil-Stuffed Zucchini Boats

Preparation Time: 35 minutes

Cooking time: 45 minutes

Servings: 2

Ingredients

Two medium zucchini halved lengthwise and seeded

2¼ cups water, divided

1 cup of rinsed dried green or red lentils

Two teaspoons olive oil

⅓ cup diced onion

Two tablespoons tomato paste

½ teaspoon oregano

¼ teaspoon garlic powder

Pinch salt

¼ cup grated part-skim mozzarella cheese

Directions:

Preheat the oven to 375°F. Line a baking sheet with parchment paper. Place the zucchini, hollow sides up, on the baking sheet, and set aside.

Bring 2 cups of water to a boil over high heat and add the lentils in a medium saucepan. Reduce the heat to low, cover, and simmer for 20 to 25 minutes.

Drain and set aside. Heat the olive oil in a medium skillet over medium-low heat. Sauté the onions until they are translucent, about 4 minutes.

Reduce the heat to low and add the cooked lentils, tomato paste, oregano, garlic powder, and salt. Add the last quarter cup of water and simmer for 3 minutes, until the liquid reduces and forms a sauce. Remove from heat.

Stuff each zucchini half with the lentil mixture, dividing it evenly, top with cheese, bake for 25 minutes and serve. The zucchini should be fork-tender, and the cheese should be melted.

Nutrition:

Calories 479

Total Fat: 9g

Carbohydrates: 74g

Protein: 31g

Baked Eggplant Parmesan

Preparation Time: 15 minutes

Cooking time: 35 minutes

Servings: 3-4

Ingredients

One small to medium eggplant, cut into ¼-inch slices

½ teaspoon salt-free Italian seasoning blend

One tablespoon olive oil

¼ cup diced onion

½ cup diced yellow or red bell pepper

Two garlic cloves, pressed or minced

1 (8-ounce) can tomato sauce

3 ounces fresh mozzarella, cut into six pieces

One tablespoon grated Parmesan cheese, divided

5 to 6 fresh basil leaves, chopped

Directions:

Preheat an oven-style air fryer to 400°F. Working in two batches, place the eggplant slices onto the air-fryer tray, and sprinkle them with Italian seasoning.

Bake for 7 minutes. Repeat with the remaining pieces, then set them aside on a plate.

In a medium skillet, heat the oil over medium heat and sauté the onion and peppers until softened about 5 minutes. Add the garlic and sauté for 1 to 2 more minutes. Add the tomato sauce and stir to combine. Remove the sauce from the heat.

Spray a 9-by-6-inch casserole dish with cooking spray. Spread one-third of the sauce into the bottom of the dish—layer eggplant slices onto the sauce.

Sprinkle with half of the Parmesan cheese. Continue layering the sauce and eggplant, ending with the sauce. Place the mozzarella pieces on the top.

Sprinkle the remaining Parmesan evenly over the entire dish. Bake in the oven for 20 minutes. Garnish with fresh basil, cut into four servings, and serve.

Nutrition:

Calories 213;

Total Fat: 12g;

Carbohydrates: 20g;

Protein: 10g

Summer Barley Pilaf with Yogurt Dill Sauce

Preparation Time: 15 minutes

Cooking Time: 30 minutes

Servings: 2-3

Ingredients:

2⅔ cups low-sodium vegetable broth

Two teaspoons avocado oil

One small zucchini, diced

⅓ cup slivered almonds

Two scallions, sliced, white and green parts separated

1 cup barley

½ cup plain nonfat Greek yogurt

Two teaspoons grated lemon zest

¼ teaspoon dried dill

Directions

In a large saucepan, bring the broth to a boil. While the broth is coming to a boil, heat the oil in a skillet. Add the zucchini and sauté 3 to 4 minutes.

Add the almonds and the white parts of the scallions and sauté for 2 minutes. Remove the mixture from the skillet and transfer it to a small bowl.

Add the barley to the skillet and sauté for 2 to 3 minutes to toast. Transfer the barley to the boiling broth and reduce the heat to low, cover, and simmer for 25 minutes or until tender.

Remove from the heat and let stand for 10 minutes, or until the liquid is absorbed.

While the barley is cooking, in a small bowl, stir together the yogurt, lemon zest, and dill and set aside.

Fluff the barley with a fork. Add the zucchini, almond, and onion mixture and mix gently.

To serve, divide the pilaf between two bowls and drizzle the yogurt over each bowl.

Nutrition:

Calories 545

Total fat: 15g

Carbohydrates: 87g

Protein: 21g

Lentil Quinoa Gratin with Butternut Squash

Preparation Time: 10 minutes

Cooking time: 1 hour, 15 minutes

Servings: 2-3

Ingredients

For the Lentils and Squash

Nonstick cooking spray

2 cups of water

½ cup dried green or red lentils, rinsed

Pinch salt

One teaspoon olive oil, divided

½ cup quinoa

¼ cup diced shallot

2 cups frozen cubed butternut squash

¼ cup low-fat milk

One teaspoon chopped fresh rosemary

Freshly ground black pepper

For the Gratin Topping

¼ cup panko bread crumbs or other bread crumbs

One teaspoon olive oil

⅓ cup shredded Gruyère cheese

Directions:

To Make the Lentils and Squash

Preheat the oven to 400°F. Spray a 1½-quart casserole dish or an 8-by-8-inch baking dish with cooking spray.

In a medium saucepan, stir together the water, lentils, and salt and bring to a boil over medium-high heat. Once the water is boiling, reduce the heat to low, cover, and simmer for 20 to 25 minutes. Then drain and transfer the lentils to a large bowl and set aside in the same saucepan, heat ½ teaspoon of oil over medium heat. Add the quinoa and quickly stir for 1 minute to toast it lightly. Cook according to the package directions, about 20 minutes.

While the quinoa cooks, heat the remaining olive oil in a medium skillet over medium-low heat, add the shallots and sauté them until they are translucent about 3 minutes.

Add the squash, milk, and rosemary and cook for 1 to 2 minutes. Remove from the heat and transfer to the lentil bowl. Add in the quinoa and gently toss all together.

Season with pepper to taste. Transfer the mixture to the casserole dish.

In a small bowl, mix the panko bread crumbs with the olive oil.

Sprinkle the bread crumbs evenly over the casserole and top them with the cheese.

Bake the casserole for 25 minutes and serve.

Nutrition:

Calories 576

Total fat: 15g

Carbohydrates: 87g

Protein: 28g

Brown Rice Casserole with Cottage Cheese

Preparation Time: 10 minutes

Cooking time: 45 minutes

Servings: 2-3

Ingredients

Nonstick cooking spray

1 cup quick-cooking brown rice

One teaspoon olive oil

½ cup diced sweet onion

1 (10-ounce) bag of fresh spinach

1½ cups low-fat cottage cheese

One tablespoon grated Parmesan cheese

¼ cup sunflower seed kernels

Directions:

Preheat the oven to 375°F. Spray a small 1½-quart casserole dish with cooking spray. Cook the rice according to the package directions. Set aside.

 Heat the oil in a large nonstick skillet over medium-low heat. Add the onion and sauté for 3 to 4 minutes. Add the spinach and cover the skillet, cooking for 1 to 2 minutes until the spinach wilts. Remove the skillet from the heat.

In a medium bowl, mix the rice, spinach mixture, and cottage cheese. Transfer the mixture to the prepared casserole dish.

Top with the Parmesan cheese and sunflower seeds, bake for 25 minutes until lightly browned, and serve.

Nutrition:

Calories 334

Total fat: 9g

Carbohydrates: 47g

Fiber: 5g

Protein: 19g

Quinoa-Stuffed Peppers

Preparation Time: 10 minutes

Cooking time: 35 minutes

Servings: 2

Ingredients

Two large green bell peppers halved

1½ teaspoons olive oil, divided

½ cup quinoa

½ cup minced onion

One garlic clove, pressed or minced

1 cup chopped portobello mushrooms

Three tablespoons grated Parmesan cheese, divided

4 ounces tomato sauce

Direction:

Preheat the oven to 400°F. Line a baking sheet with parchment paper. Place the pepper halves on the baking sheet.

Brush the insides of peppers with ½ teaspoon olive oil and bake for 10 minutes. Remove the baking sheet from the oven and set aside.

While the peppers bake, cook the quinoa in a large saucepan over medium heat according to the package directions and set aside.

Heat the remaining oil in a medium-size skillet over medium heat. Add the onion and sauté until it's translucent about 3 minutes. Add the garlic and cook for 1 minute. Add the mushrooms to the skillet, reduce the heat to medium-low, cover, and cook for 5 to 6 minutes or until the mushrooms are tender. Uncover, and if there's still liquid in the pan, reduce the heat and cook until the liquid evaporates.

Add the mushroom mixture, one tablespoon of Parmesan, and the tomato sauce to the quinoa and gently stir to combine.

Carefully spoon the quinoa mixture into each pepper half and sprinkle with the remaining Parmesan.

Return the peppers to the oven, bake for 10 to 15 more minutes until tender, and serve.

Nutrition:

Calories 292

Total fat: 9g

Carbohydrates: 45g

Fiber: 8g

Protein: 12g

Black Bean Burgers

Preparation Time: 15 minutes

Cooking time: 20 minutes

Servings: 4

Ingredients

½ cup quick-cooking brown rice

Two teaspoons canola oil, divided

½ cup finely chopped carrots

¼ cup finely chopped onion

1 (15-ounce) can black beans, drained and rinsed

One tablespoon salt-free mesquite seasoning blend

Four small, hard rolls

Directions:

Cook the rice according to the package directions and set aside. Heat 1 teaspoon of oil in a large nonstick skillet over medium heat. Add the carrots and onions and cook until the onions are translucent about 4 minutes.

Reduce the heat to low, cover, and continue cooking for 5 to 6 minutes, until the carrots are tender. Add the beans and seasoning to the skillet and continue cooking for 2 to 3 more minutes.

Transfer the bean mixture to a food processor and wipe the skillet clean. Pulse the bean mixture 3 to 4 times or until the mixture is coarsely blended. Transfer the mixture to a medium bowl and fold in the brown rice until well combined.

Divide the mixture evenly and form it into four patties with your hands. Heat the remaining oil in the skillet. Cook the patties for 4 to 5 minutes per side, turning once.

Serve the burgers on the rolls with your choice of toppings.

Nutrition

Calories: 368

Total fat: 6g

Carbohydrates: 66g

Fiber: 8g;

Protein: 13g

DASH-Style Cobb Salad

Preparation Time: 20 minutes

Cooking time: 15 minutes

Servings: 2

Ingredients

1 (6-ounce) skinless, boneless chicken breast

Zest and juice of 1 lemon

Two tablespoons white wine vinegar

One tablespoon extra-virgin olive oil

One tablespoon sweet onion, minced

½ teaspoon Dijon mustard

One head romaine lettuce, roughly chopped

One large hardboiled egg, sliced

Four plum tomatoes, sliced

One avocado, thinly sliced

1-ounce blue cheese crumbles

One tablespoon roasted sunflower seeds

Directions:

To poach the chicken, fill large saucepan three-quarters full of water and bring it to a boil over high heat. Add the zest or rind from half of the lemon to the water. Add the chicken, reduce the heat to low, cover, and simmer for about 10 minutes.

The chicken should be opaque and white in the center. If it's showing any pink, continue simmering for another 5 minutes. Remove the saucepan from the heat and take the chicken out to cool.

While the chicken is cooking, mix the dressing. Combine the vinegar, lemon juice, oil, onion, and mustard in a small bowl or jar and mix thoroughly.

Divide the lettuce between two plates and top it with the egg, tomato, and avocado slices.

Cut the chicken into ⅛-inch thick slices and add it to the salads. Drizzle the salads with the dressing, top them with blue cheese crumbles and sunflower seeds, and serve.

Nutritions:

Calories: 542

Total Fat: 34g

Carbohydrates: 31g

Fiber: 17g

Protein: 35g

High Protein Spring Mix with Tuna & Egg

Preparation Time: 15 minutes

Cooking time: 30 minutes

Servings: 2

Ingredients:

2 (2.6-ounce) pouches of albacore tuna

Two large hardboiled eggs, chopped

¼ cup chopped celery

Two tablespoons minced onion

Two tablespoons plain Greek yogurt

One tablespoon mayonnaise

¼ teaspoon dried dill

4 cups spring mix or other salad greens

1 cup grape tomatoes, halved

½ cup finely chopped yellow bell peppers

One tablespoon extra-virgin olive oil

One tablespoon apple cider vinegar

Direction:

In a medium bowl, mix the tuna, eggs, celery, onion, yogurt, mayonnaise, and dill until well combined. Divide the spring mix between two plates. Add half of the tomatoes and peppers to each plate and dress the salads with oil and vinegar.

Top each of the salads with a large scoop of the tuna mixture and serve.

Nutrition:

Calories: 370

Total Fat: 20g

Carbohydrates: 23g

Fiber: 4g

Protein: 27g

Arugula Salad with Tuna & Roasted Peppers

Preparation Time: 15 minutes

Cooking time: 21 minutes

Servings: 2

Ingredients:

Two tablespoons plus one teaspoon olive oil, divided

Two tablespoons balsamic vinegar

Juice of 1½ lemons, divided

Two tuna steaks (4 to 6 ounces each)

4 to 6 mini bell peppers, seeded and halved lengthwise

4 cups arugula

¼ cup fresh basil, chopped

Freshly ground black pepper

One mango, diced

Lemon quarters, for garnish

Directions:
Preheat the grill to 450°F.

Mix 1 tablespoon of the olive oil, the balsamic vinegar, and the juice of half a lemon in a shallow bowl. Add the tuna to the bowl and marinate it while the peppers cook.

Place the peppers on a small grill pan, then put it on the hot grill. Grill for 10 to 15 minutes, or until the peppers are slightly charred, turning occasionally.

Transfer them to a small bowl. Using kitchen shears, chop the peppers into large pieces. Add one teaspoon of olive oil and set aside to cool.

Place the tuna steaks on the hot grill and grill for 3 minutes per side for medium doneness (discard the marinade). Remove the fish from the grill and cut each steak into ¼-inch slices. Cover the tuna with foil to keep it warm.

If you do not have a grill, roast the peppers on a baking sheet in a 450°F oven for 25 to 40 minutes, turning them halfway through the cooking time. Cook the tuna in a large nonstick skillet over medium-high heat, 2 to 3 minutes per side.

In a medium bowl, toss together the arugula and basil. In a small bowl, mix the remaining olive oil with the remaining lemon juice. Pour the mixture over the salad and toss to coat.

Divide the arugula mixture between two plates. Season to taste with pepper. Top with the roasted peppers, mango, and tuna slices. Garnish with a lemon quarter, if desired.

Nutrition:

Calories 511

Total Fat: 23g

Carbohydrates: 50g

Fiber: 6g

Protein: 32g

Bold Bean Shrimp Fiesta Salad

Preparation Time: 20 minutes

Cooking time: 0 minutes

Servings: 2

Ingredients:

2 cups frozen corn, thawed

1 cup canned black beans, drained and rinsed

1 cup chopped cooked shrimp

1 cup halved grape tomatoes

One jalapeño pepper, seeded and diced

Two tablespoons diced red onion

Juice of 2 limes

¼ cup chopped fresh cilantro

1½ tablespoons olive oil

⅛ teaspoon salt

Pinch freshly ground black pepper

Directions:

In a medium bowl, combine the corn, beans, shrimp, tomatoes, jalapeño, and onion. In a small bowl or jar, mix the lime juice, cilantro, olive oil, salt, and pepper. Add the dressing to the corn and bean mixture, toss until combined, and serve.

Nutrition: 422

Total Fat: 13g

Carbohydrates: 68g;

Fiber: 14g

Protein: 19g

Salmon-Topped Spinach Salad with Avocado

Preparation Time: 20 minutes

Cooking time: 10 minutes

Servings: 2

Ingredients:

Two tablespoons avocado oil

Juice of 1 lime

One tablespoon plus ½ teaspoon mesquite salt-free seasoning blend (or any salt-free seasoning), divided

Two salmon fillets (4 ounces each)

3 cups fresh baby spinach, washed and stemmed

¼ cup dried cranberries

1½ tablespoons sunflower seeds

One avocado, sliced

Directions:
Preheat an oven-style air fryer to 350°F, on the air-fry setting. In a small jar or bowl, mix the avocado oil, lime juice, and ½ teaspoon of the mesquite seasoning. Set aside.

Rub both sides of each salmon fillet with the remaining mesquite seasoning and air-fry for 10 minutes. While the salmon is air-frying, in a medium bowl, toss the spinach with the cranberries and sunflower seeds. Drizzle the salad with the dressing and toss to combine.

Divide the spinach mixture between two plates. Top each salad with the avocado and the salmon and serve.

Nutrition:

Calories: 568

Total Fat: 40g

Carbohydrates: 29g

Fiber: 11g

Protein: 28g

Chapter 26: Anti- Hypertension Side Dishes

Steamed Asparagus With Horseradish Dip

Preparation Time: 5 minutes

Cooking Time: 15 minutes

Servings: 6-12

Ingredients:

32 fresh asparagus spears (trimmed)

1/4 cup Parmesan cheese (grated)

1 cup mayonnaise (reduced-fat)

1/2 teaspoon Worcestershire sauce

One tablespoon prepared horseradish

Directions:

Place the asparagus in a steamer. Steam for 4 minutes. Immediately transfer the asparagus in ice water. Drain. Pat with paper towels to dry.

In a bowl, mix the rest of the ingredients.

Serve the asparagus with the dip.

Nutrition:

Calories: 63

Carbohydrates: 3 g

Fat: 5 g

Protein: 1 g

Mint, Lime, And Grapefruit Yogurt Parfait

Preparation Time: 15 minutes

Cooking Time: 0 minutes

Servings: 1

Ingredients:

4 cups reduced-fat plain yogurt

Four large red grapefruit

Three tablespoons honey

Two tablespoons lime juice

Two teaspoons lime zest (grated)

Fresh mint leaves (torn)

Directions

Cut off the peel the grapefruit, including the outer membrane. Slice following the membrane on each segment to remove the fruit inside.

In a bowl, mix well the lime zest, yogurt, and lime juice—layer into six parfait glasses the half of the grapefruit. The next layer is half of the yogurt mixture. Repeat the layers.

Top each parfait glass with honey and mint. Serve.

Nutrition:

Calories: 207

Carbohydrates: 39 g

Fat: 3 g

Protein: 10 g

Pita Chips With Hummus Dip

Preparation Time: 15 minutes

Cooking Time: 0 minutes

Servings: 3-6

Ingredients:

One 10-ounce carton hummus

1 cup feta cheese (crumbled)

1/2 cup Greek olives (chopped)

1/4 cup red onion (finely chopped)

One large English cucumber (chopped)

Two medium tomatoes (seeded, chopped)

Baked pita chips

Directions:

In a shallow round dish, spread the hummus evenly. Layer with onion, tomatoes, olives, cucumber, and cheese. Chill in the fridge for an hour or more. Serve with chips.

Nutrition:

Calories: 88

Carbohydrates: 6 g

Fat: 5 g

Protein: 4 g

Almond And Fruit Bites

Preparation Time: 40 minutes + chilling

Cooking Time: 0 minutes

Servings: 1

Ingredients:

3 3/4 cups sliced almonds (divided)

2 cups dried apricots (finely chopped)

1 cup pistachios(finely chopped, toasted)

1 cup dried cherries (finely chopped)

1/4 cup honey

1/4 teaspoon almond extract

Directions:

In a food processor, pulse the 1 1/4 cups of almonds until chopped finely. Transfer to a shallow bowl for coating later. Put in the rest of the almonds into the food processor. Pulse until chopped finely. Add in the almond extract. While pulsing, add the honey gradually. Transfer to a bowl. Stir in the cherries and apricots.

Divide the dough into six parts. Roll each portion into 1/2-inch thick logs. Wrap each log in plastic. Chill in the fridge for an hour to firm. Unwrap each log. Slice into one 1/2-inch piece. Roll half of the bites in pistachios. Roll the other half in almonds. Serve or store in airtight containers.

Nutrition:

Calories: 86

Carbohydrates: 10 g

Fat: 5 g

Protein: 2 g

Banana Split—Dash Diet Style

Preparation Time: 10 minutes

Cooking Time: 0 minutes

Servings: 1/4 of the dish

Ingredients:

Four small bananas (peeled, halved lengthwise)

1 cup fresh raspberries

2 cups fat-free vanilla Greek yogurt

1/2 cup granola without raisins

Two small peaches (sliced)

Two tablespoons sunflower kernels

Two tablespoons sliced almonds (toasted)

Two tablespoons honey

Directions:

Equally, portion the bananas among four dishes. Top with the rest of the ingredients. Serve.

Nutrition:

Calories: 340

Carbohydrates: 61 g

Fat: 6 g

Protein: 17 g

Chai Almond Granola

Preparation Time: 20 minutes

Cooking Time: 1 1/4 hours

Serving: 1/2 cup

Ingredients:

3 cups quick-cooking oats

1 cup shredded coconut (sweetened)

2 cups almonds (coarsely chopped)

1/2 cup honey

1/3 cup sugar

1/4 cup boiling water

1/4 cup olive oil

Two chai tea bags

Two teaspoons vanilla extract

3/4 teaspoon ground cinnamon

3/4 teaspoon salt

1/4 teaspoon ground cardamom

3/4 teaspoon ground nutmeg

Directions:

Preheat oven to 250 degrees Fahrenheit. Grease a rimmed baking pan.

Steep the tea bags for 5 minutes in boiling water.

In a bowl, mix well the coconut, almonds, and oats.

Discard the tea bags. Mix well the rest of the ingredients into the tea. Pour the tea mixture into the oat mixture. Mix well.

Spread out the mixture evenly on the greased baking pan.

Bake for 1 1/4 hours, stirring every 20 minutes.

Cool completely. Serve or store in an airtight container.

Nutrition:

Calories: 272

Carbohydrates: 29 g

Fat: 16 g

Protein: 6 g

Almond Butter And Chocolate Bites

Preparation Time: 5 minutes

Cooking Time: 0 minutes

Serving Size: 1 teaspoon almond butter and two 1/4-ounce squares chocolate

Ingredients:

Four teaspoons almond butter

Eight 1/4-ounce squares bittersweet chocolate

Directions:

Spread 1/2 teaspoon of almond butter on each chocolate square. Serve.

Nutrition:

Calories: 79

Carbohydrates: 9.4 g

Fat: 5.8 g

Protein: 1.2 g

Hummus And Vegetables Sandwich

Preparation Time: 10 minutes

Cooking Time: 0 minutes

Servings: 1

Ingredients:

Three tablespoons hummus

Two slices whole-grain bread

1/2 cup mixed salad greens

1/4 cup carrot (shredded)

1/4 cup cucumber (sliced)

1/4 avocado (mashed)

1/4 medium red bell pepper (sliced)

Directions:

Spread the hummus on a slice of bread.

Spread the avocado on the other slice of bread.

Fill the sandwich with the rest of the ingredients.

Slice in half. Serve.

Nutrition:

Calories: 325

Carbohydrates: 39.7 g

Fat: 14.3 g

Protein: 12.8 g

Banana Peanut Butter Cinnamon Toast

Preparation Time: 5 minutes

Cooking Time: 0 minutes

Serving Size: 1 toast

Ingredients:

One small banana (sliced)

One tablespoon peanut butter

One slice whole-wheat bread (toasted)

Cinnamon (to taste)

Directions:

Spread the peanut butter on the toast. Arrange the banana slices on top.

Garnish with cinnamon. Serve.

Nutrition:

Calories: 266

Carbohydrates: 38.3 g

Fat: 9.3 g

Protein: 8.1 g

Oat With Peanut Butter Energy Balls

Preparation Time: 15 minutes

Cooking Time: 15 minutes

Servings: 1

Ingredients:

1/4 cup natural peanut butter

1/2 cup rolled oats

3/4 cup Medjool dates (chopped)

Chia seeds (for garnish)

Directions:

In a bowl with hot water, soak the dates for 10 minutes. Drain.

In a food processor, put in the oats, dates, and peanut butter. Proccss until chopped finely.

Roll the mixture into 12 balls. Garnish with chia seeds.

Chill in the fridge for an hour or more. Serve.

Nutrition:

Calories: 73

Carbohydrates: 10.1 g

Fat: 3 g

Protein: 1.8 g

Cabbage Rolls

Preparation Time: 15 minutes

Cooking Time: 20 minutes

Servings: 1 1/3 cups and 2/3 cup rice

Ingredients:

One 28-ounce can whole plum tomatoes (undrained)

One 8-ounce can tomato sauce

One pound extra-lean ground beef (95% lean)

One large onion (chopped)

One medium green pepper (thin strips)

One small head cabbage (sliced thinly)

4 cups brown rice (hot cooked)

Two tablespoons cider vinegar

One tablespoon brown sugar

One teaspoon dried thyme (seasoning)

One teaspoon dried oregano (seasoning)

1/2 teaspoon pepper (seasoning)

Directions:

Drain the tomatoes. Set aside the liquid. Chop the tomatoes coarsely.

In a skillet over medium heat, cook the onion and beef for 8 minutes.

Add in the vinegar, tomato sauce, seasonings, brown sugar, tomatoes, and reserved liquid.

Stir in the cabbage and pepper. Cover. Cook for 6 minutes with occasional stirring. Uncover. Cook for another 8 minutes. Serve with rice.

Nutrition:

Calories: 332

Carbohydrates: 50 g

Fat: 5 g

Protein: 22 g

Pinto Beans Salad With Rice

Preparation Time: 10 minutes

Cooking Time: 20 minutes

Servings: 1/4 part of the dish

Ingredients:

One 8.8-ounce package ready-to-serve brown rice

1 15-ounce can pinto beans (rinsed, drained)

One 4-ounce can green chilies (chopped)

1 cup of frozen corn

1/4 cup fresh cilantro (chopped)

1/2 cup salsa

1/4 cup cheddar cheese (shredded finely)

One tablespoon olive oil

1 1/2 teaspoons ground cumin

1 1/2 teaspoons chili powder

One small onion (chopped)

One bunch romaine (4 wedges)

Two garlic cloves (minced)

Directions:

In a skillet over medium heat, heat the oil. Sautee the onion and corn for 5 minutes.

Add the cumin, chili powder, and garlic—sautee for 1 minute more.

Add the cilantro, salsa, green chilies, rice, and pinto beans. Cook until heated through with occasional stirring.

Put the romaine wedges in a bowl. Pour the pinto bean mixture over the wedges. Garnish with cheese. Serve.

Nutrition:

Calories: 331

Carbohydrates: 50 g

Fat: 8 g

Protein: 12 g

Cauliflower Steak Curry With Tzatziki Sauce And Red Rice

Preparation Time: 30 minutes

Cooking Time: 30 minutes

Serving: 1 cauliflower steak, 3/4 cup rice, and 1/4 cup tzatziki sauce

Ingredients:

Tzatziki Sauce:

1/4 cup sour cream

3/4 cup plain Greek yogurt (nonfat)

One clove garlic (minced)

One tablespoon lemon juice

1/2 medium cucumber (seeded, grated)

1/2 teaspoon kosher salt

Cauliflower Steaks and Rice:

1/3 cup extra-virgin olive oil

1 cup red rice

Two tablespoons fresh cilantro (chopped)

One tablespoon lemon juice

Two medium heads cauliflower

1/2 teaspoon kosher salt

Two teaspoons curry powder

Directions:

Tzatziki Sauce:

In a bowl, whisk the sour cream, yogurt, garlic, lemon juice, and salt until smooth. Fold in the cucumber. Chill in the fridge.

Cauliflower and Rice:

Preheat oven to 450 degrees Fahrenheit. Line a rimmed baking tray with foil.

Cook rice according to package instructions. Keep warm.

In a bowl, whisk well the lemon juice, oil, salt, and curry powder.

Discard the outer leaves of the cauliflower. Keep the stems intact.

Make four cauliflower steaks. They should be 1-inch thick slices from the center of each cauliflower head down to the stem.

Cut the rest of the cauliflower into 3/4-inch florets.

Place the steaks and florets on the lined baking tray in a single layer. Brush all sides of the cauliflower with the curry mixture.

Roast for 35 minutes, turning halfway.

Store 6 tablespoons of tzatziki sauce and florets in the fridge for another recipe.

Equally, divide the cooked rice among four plates. Top each rice with steak, 1/4 cup of tzatziki sauce. Garnish with cilantro. Serve.

Nutrition:

Calories: 410

Carbohydrates: 48.5 g

Fat: 21.3 g

Barley Vegetable And Turkey Soup

Preparation Time: 5 minutes

Cooking Time: 25 minutes

Servings: 1 1/3 cups

Ingredients:

6 cups chicken broth (reduced-sodium)

2 cups fresh baby spinach

2 cups cooked turkey breast (cubed)

2/3 cup quick-cooking barley

One medium onion (chopped)

Five medium carrots (chopped)

One tablespoon canola oil

1/2 teaspoon pepper

Directions:

In a saucepan over medium heat, heat the oil. Sautee the onion and carrots for 5 minutes.

Stir in the broth and barley. Bring to a boil.

Lower the heat. Cover. Simmer for 15 minutes.

Add the spinach, turkey, and pepper. Stir. Cook until heated. Serve.

Nutrition:

Calories: 208

Carbohydrates: 23 g

Fat: 4 g

Protein: 21 g

Grilled Steak Salad (Southwestern Style)

Preparation Time: 25 minutes

Cooking Time: 20 minutes

Servings: 2 ounces beef and 2 cups pasta mixture

Ingredients:

One 3/4-pound beef top sirloin steak (1 inch thick)

Two large ears sweet corn (husks removed)

Three poblano peppers (halved, seeded)

One large sweet onion (1/2-inch rings)

Two large tomatoes

2 cups multigrain bow tie pasta (uncooked)

One tablespoon olive oil

1/4 teaspoon ground cumin

1/4 teaspoon salt

1/4 teaspoon pepper

Dressing:

1/3 cup fresh cilantro (chopped)

1/4 cup lime juice

1/4 teaspoon salt

One tablespoon olive oil

1/4 teaspoon pepper

1/4 teaspoon ground cumin

Directions:

Rub the steak with pepper, cumin, and salt.

Brush oil on the onion, corn, and poblano peppers.

Grill the steak to your desired doneness over medium heat.

Grill the oiled vegetables for 10 minutes with occasional turning.

Cook the pasta according to package instructions. Drain.

Chop the tomatoes, peppers, and onion. Remove the corn from the cob. Put them all in a bowl.

In another bowl, whisk together the oil, lime juice, cumin, salt, and pepper. Stir in the cilantro.

Add the pasta into the chopped vegetables. Pour the dressing over. Toss.

Thinly slice the steak. Add to the salad. Serve.

Nutrition:

Calories: 456

Carbohydrates: 58 g

Fat: 13 g

Protein: 30 g

Chapter 27: Anti-Hypertension Desserts Recipes

Honey Ricotta with Espresso and Chocolate Chips

Preparation time: 5 minutes

Cooking time: 15 minutes

Servings: 2

Ingredients:

8 ounces ricotta cheese

Two tablespoons honey

Two tablespoons espresso, chilled or room temperature

One teaspoon dark chocolate chips or chocolate shavings

Directions:

in a medium bowl, whip together the ricotta cheese and honey until light and smooth, 4 to 5 minutes.

Spoon the ricotta cheese–honey mixture evenly into two dessert bowls. Drizzle 1-tablespoon espresso into each dish and sprinkle with chocolate chips or shavings.

Nutrition:

Calories: 235

Total fat: 10g

Total carbohydrates: 25g

Protein: 13g

Roasted Plums with Nut Crumble

Preparation time: 5 minutes

Cooking time: 25 minutes

Servings: 4

Ingredients:

¼ cup honey

¼ cup freshly squeezed orange juice

Four large plums halved and pitted

¼ cup whole-wheat pastry flour

One tablespoon pure maple sugar

One tablespoon nuts, coarsely chopped (your choice like almonds, pecans, and walnuts)

1½ teaspoons canola oil

½ cup plain greek yogurt

Directions:

preheat the oven to 400°f. Combine the honey and orange juice in a square baking dish. Place the plums, cut-side down, in the dish. Roast about 15 minutes, and then turn the plums over and roast an additional 10 minutes, or until tender and juicy.

In a medium bowl, combine the flour, maple sugar, nuts, and canola oil and mix well. Spread on a small baking sheet and bake alongside the plums, tossing once, until golden brown, about 5 minutes. Set aside until the plums have finished cooking.

Serve the plums drizzled with pan juices and topped with the nut crumble and a dollop of yogurt.

Nutrition:

Calories: 175

Total fat: 3g

Total carbohydrates: 36g

Protein: 4g

Figs with Mascarpone and Honey

Preparation time: 5 minutes

Cooking time: 5 minutes

Servings: 4

Ingredients:

⅓ cup walnuts, chopped

Eight fresh figs halved

¼ cup mascarpone cheese

One tablespoon honey

¼ teaspoon flaked sea salt

Directions:

In a large pan, put it over medium heat, toast the walnuts, often stirring, 3 to 5 minutes.

Arrange the figs cut-side up on a plate or platter. Using your finger, make a small depression in each fig's cut side and fill with mascarpone cheese. Sprinkle with a bit of the walnut, drizzle with the honey, and add a tiny pinch of sea salt.

Nutrition:

Calories: 200g

Total fat: 13g

Total carbohydrates: 24g

Protein: 3g

Greek Yogurt Chocolate "Mousse" With Berries

Preparation time: 30 minutes

Cooking time: 0 minutes

Servings: 4

Ingredients:

2 cups plain Greek yogurt

¼ cup heavy cream

¼ cup pure maple syrup

Three tablespoons unsweetened cocoa powder

Two teaspoons vanilla extract

¼ teaspoon kosher salt

1 cup fresh mixed berries

¼ cup of chocolate chips

Directions:

Place the yogurt, cream, maple syrup, cocoa powder, vanilla, salt in the bowl of a stand mixer, or use a large bowl with an electric hand mixer. Mix at medium-high speed until fluffy, about 5 minutes.

Spoon evenly among four bowls and put in the refrigerator to set for at least 15 minutes.

Serve each bowl with ¼ cup mixed berries and one tablespoon chocolate chips.

Nutrition:

calories: 300g;

Total fat: 11g

Total carbohydrates: 35g

Protein: 16g

Individual Meringues with Strawberries, Mint, and Toasted Coconut

Preparation time: 25 minutes

Cooking time: 1 hour, 30 minutes

Servings: 6

Ingredients:

Four large egg whites

One teaspoon vanilla extract

½ teaspoon cream of tartar

¾ cup of sugar

8 ounces strawberries, diced

¼ cup fresh mint, chopped

¼ cup unsweetened shredded coconut, toasted

Directions:

Preheat the oven to 225°f. Line 2 baking sheets with parchment paper.

Place the egg whites, vanilla, and cream of tartar in the bowl of a stand mixer (or use a large bowl with an electric hand mixer); beat at medium speed until soft peaks form, about 2 to 3 minutes. Put it on high speed and gradually add the sugar, beating until stiff peaks form and the mixture looks shiny and smooth about 2 to 3 minutes.

Using a spatula or spoon, drop ⅓ cup of meringue onto a prepared baking sheet, smooth out and make shapelier as desired. In total, make 12 dollops, 6 per sheet, leaving at least 1 inch between dollops.

Bake for 1½ hours, rotating baking sheets between top and bottom, front and back, halfway through. After 1½ hours, turn off the oven, but keep the door closed. Leave the meringues in the oven for an additional 30 minutes. You can leave the meringues in the oven even longer (or overnight), or you may let them finish cooling to room temperature.

Combine the strawberries, mint, and coconut in a medium bowl. Serve two meringues per person topped with the fruit mixture.

Nutrition :

Calories: 150g

Total fat: 2g

Total carbohydrates: 29g

Protein: 3g

Pistachio-Stuffed Dates

Preparation time: 10 minutes

Cooking time: 0 minute

Servings: 4

Ingredients:

½ cup unsalted pistachios shelled

¼ teaspoon kosher salt

Eight Medjool dates pitted

Directions:

Add the pistachios and salt in a food processor. Process until combined to chunky nut butter, 3 to 5 minutes.

Split open the dates and spoon the pistachio nut butter into each half.

Nutrition:

Calories: 220g

Total fat: 7g

Total carbohydrates: 41g

Protein: 4g

Tzatziki

Preparation time: 10 minutes

Cooking time: 0 minutes

Servings: 1½ cups

Ingredients:

Two Persian cucumbers or ½ hothouse or English cucumber

1 cup plain greek yogurt

Two tablespoons fresh dill, chopped

Two tablespoons fresh mint, chopped

Two tablespoons lemon juice

One tablespoon extra-virgin olive oil

One garlic clove, minced

½ teaspoon kosher salt

Directions:

Using a box grater, grate the cucumbers. In a medium bowl, combine the grated cucumbers, yogurt, dill, mint, lemon juice, olive oil, garlic, and salt; mix well.

Nutrition:

Calories: 45g

Total fat: 0g

Total carbohydrates: 3g

protein: 3g

Salsa Verde

Preparation time: 5 minutes

Cooking time: 0 minute

Servings: 1

Ingredients:

2 cups parsley

¼ cup lemon juice

Two teaspoons capers, rinsed

Four anchovies, chopped

½ teaspoon kosher salt

¼ teaspoon freshly ground black pepper

½ cup extra-virgin olive oil

Directions:

Add the parsley, lemon juice, capers, anchovies, salt, and black pepper to a food processor. Process until minced. Next, add the olive oil and process until it reaches your desired consistency. Refrigerate until ready to use. Any leftovers can store in an airtight container for up to 1 week.

Nutrition:

Calories: 130g

Total fat: 14g

Total carbohydrates: 2g

Protein: 1g

Lemon Tahini Dressing

Preparation time: 5 minutes

Cooking time: 0 minute

Servings: ½ cup

Ingredients:

¼ cup tahini

Three tablespoons lemon juice

Three tablespoons warm water

¼ teaspoon kosher salt

¼ teaspoon pure maple syrup

⅛ teaspoon cayenne pepper

¼ teaspoon ground cumin

Directions:

Whisk together the tahini, lemon juice, water, salt, maple syrup, cumin, and cayenne pepper until smooth in a medium bowl.

Nutrition:

calories: 90g

Total fat: 7g

Total carbohydrates: 5g

Protein: 3g

Yogurt Tahini Dressing

Preparation time: 5 minutes

Cooking time: 0 minute

Servings:1

Ingredients:

½ cup plain greek yogurt

⅓ cup tahini

¼ cup freshly squeezed orange juice

½ teaspoon kosher salt

Direction:

First. You have to mix the tahini, salt, orange juice, and yogurt until smooth in a medium bowl. Place in the refrigerator until ready to serve.

Nutrition:

calories: 70g

total fat: 2g

Total carbohydrates: 4g

Protein: 4g

Lemon Vinaigrette

Preparation time: 5 minutes

Cooking time: 0 minutes

Servings: 1

Ingredients:

¼ cup lemon juice

¼ cup white wine vinegar

Two tablespoons shallot, minced

Two teaspoons dijon mustard

½ teaspoon honey

½ teaspoon kosher salt

¼ teaspoon freshly ground black pepper

½ cup extra-virgin olive oil

Directions:

Mix the lemon juice, vinegar, shallot, mustard, honey, salt, and black pepper in a medium bowl,. Add the olive oil and whisk well.

Nutrition:

Calories: 125

Total fat: 14g

Total carbohydrates: 1g

Protein: 0g

Olive Mint Vinaigrette

Preparation time: 5 minutes

Cooking time: 0 minute

Servings: 1

Ingredients:

¼ cup white wine vinegar

¼ teaspoon honey

¼ teaspoon kosher salt

¼ teaspoon freshly ground black pepper

¼ cup extra-virgin olive oil

¼ cup olives, pitted and minced

Two tablespoons fresh mint, minced

Directions:

Mix the honey, vinegar, black pepper, and salt in a bowl. Add the olive oil and whisk well. Add the olives and mint, and mix well. Store any leftovers in the refrigerator in an airtight container for up to 5 days.

Nutrition:

Calories: 135

Total Fat: 15g

Total carbohydrates: 1g

Protein: 0g

Toasted Almond Ambrosia

Cooking time: 30 minutes

Preparation time: 10 minutes

Servings: 2

Ingredients:

½ cup almonds, slivered

½ cup coconut, shredded & unsweetened

3 cups pineapple, cubed

Five oranges, segment

One banana, halved lengthwise, peeled & sliced

Two red apples, cored & diced

Two tablespoons cream sherry

Mint leaves, fresh to garnish

Directions:

Preheat your oven to 325, and then get out a baking sheet. Roast your almonds for ten minutes, making sure they're spread out evenly.

Transfer them to a plate and then toast your coconut on the same baking sheet—toast for ten minutes.

Mix your banana, sherry, oranges, apples, and pineapple in a bowl.

Divide the mixture, not serving bowls, and top with coconut and almonds.

Garnish with mint before serving.

Nutrition:

Calories: 177

Protein: 3.4 g

Fat: 4.9 g

Carbs: 36 g

Apple Dumplings

Cooking time: 40 minutes

Preparation time: 20 minutes

Servings: 4

Ingredients:

Dough:

One tablespoon butter

One teaspoon honey, raw

1 cup whole wheat flour

Two tablespoons buckwheat flour

Two tablespoons rolled oats

Two tablespoons brandy or apple liquor

Filling:

Two tablespoons honey, raw

One teaspoon nutmeg

Six tart apples, sliced thin

One lemon, zested

Directions:

Turn the oven to 350.

Get out a food processor and mix your butter, flours, honey, and oats until it forms a crumbly mixture.

Add in your brandy or apple liquor, pulsing until it forms a dough.

Seal in plastic and place it in the fridge for two hours.

Toss your apples in lemon zest, honey, and nutmeg.

Roll your dough into a sheet that's a quarter-inch thick. Cut out eight-inch circles, placing each circle into a muffin tray that has been greased.

Press the dough down and then stuff with the apple mixture. Fold the edges, and pinch them closed. Make sure that they are well sealed.

Bake for a half-hour until golden brown, and serve drizzled in honey.

Nutrition:

Calories: 178g

Protein: 5 g

Fat: 4 g

Carbs: 23 g

Apricot Biscotti

Preparation time: 15 minutes

Cooking time: 50 minutes

Servings: 4

Ingredients:

Two tablespoons honey, dark

Two tablespoons olive oil

½ teaspoon almond extract

¼ cup almonds, chopped roughly

2/3 cup apricots, dried

Two tablespoons milk, 1% & low fat

Two eggs, beaten lightly

¾ cup whole wheat flour

¾ cup all-purpose flour

¼ cup brown sugar, packed firm

One teaspoon baking powder

Directions:

Heat the oven to 350, then mix your baking powder, brown sugar, and flours in a bowl.

Whisk your canola oil, eggs, almond extract, honey, and milk. Mix well until it forms a smooth dough. Fold in the apricots and almonds.

Put your dough on plastic wrap, and then roll it out to a twelve-inch long and three-inch wide rectangle. Place this dough on a baking sheet, and bake for twenty-five minutes. It should turn golden brown. Allow it to cool, slice it to ½-inch thick slices, and then bake for another fifteen minutes. It should be crispy.

Nutrition:

Calories: 291g

Protein: 2 g

Fat: 2 g

Carbs: 12 g

Conclusion

Living with hypertension can be a stressful challenge as it is associated with several other life-threatening diseases and health problems such as heart diseases, diabetes, and renal diseases. Hypertension is also referred to as a silent killer. But diet and lifestyle changes can have a significant impact on managing these issues. DASH diet is designed with two different levels of sodium. The first level for reducing sodium in the diet was 2300 mg per day and the second level was 1500 mg, which was the ultimate target to cut down on sodium content.

The diet and physical activity alone can control prehypertension. Medication is only suggested to those at higher risk of getting a stroke or any other associated complications. Individuals who are overweight or obese are at higher risk of being affected by these health issues. Exercise and dietary modifications can help in reducing weight and controlling blood pressure.

The DASH diet allows for easy weight loss. A healthy diet, one focused on fruits, vegetables, and other main DASH foods, can allow you to fill your meals without consuming too much. And new research shows that the use of calcium-rich dairy foods in your diet can have different weight-loss benefits. Therefore,

DASH provides the perfect foundation for a weight loss strategy. Reducing weight is recommended as one of the main changes in lifestyle to help manage hypertension. Far more significant benefits can be predicted when weight loss and the DASH diet program are combined.

Evidence has shown that DASH diet foods are capable of supporting weight loss. You should fill up with a diet rich in fruits and vegetables without overdoing the calories. Lean meat, fish, and poultry contain fewer calories for satiating protein than higher-fat meats. For example, eight ounces of boiled shrimp have the same calories as three ounces of corned beef, while at the same time giving more satisfaction. Low-fat dairy products have much fewer calories than the higher versions of fat, which they substitute. And research suggests diets rich in milk calcium promote weight loss, 66 particularly with an extra fat reduction around your waist. Having your weight above the healthy weight is one of the significant risk factors for high blood pressure growth. The excess weight is even more dangerous for kids and teens.

High blood pressure parents, who follow the DASH diet, greatly help their children by providing the right food and avoiding calorie-laden meals. Through watching their parents' children learn to eat in healthy patterns. As a parent, you should model healthy behavior and help your children escape a lifetime blood pressure medication regimen.

Knowing that your decisions are essential for the whole family will motivate you to make changes in your diet and lifestyle.

There are a lot of ways to decide if your weight is optimal for you. For many years the Metropolitan Life Weight Tables were used to classify healthy weights. Recently, BMI (body mass index, showing the weight-to-height relation) has become an essential tool for beneficial weight assessment. The indicator of health (or fatness) is body fat percentage. And some healthcare professionals say a healthy weight is a weight you don't have health problems with, or at least none related to your weight. The National Institutes of Health issued new healthy weight recommendations in 1998, based on BMI. We were designed to provide information on the weight-to-height ratio of 67, associated with lower disease risk. BMI is based on a kilogram weight calculation divided by height in meters, squared. It is essential to accept that not everyone in elevated risk is at greater risk of disease. The BMI tables represent an overall risk to large numbers of people but not to individuals. For example, A sedentary person, who have a healthy weight, may have a higher risk of disease than someone who is slightly overweight but physically fit. And the BMI tables will look overweight by a football player, though he may not be overfat. BMI that is less than 19 is considered underweight, 19-25 is a healthy weight, 26-30 is overweight, 31-39 is obese, and a BMI of more than 40 is considered extremely obese. One can calculate health (or fatness) by looking at the percentage of body fat.

The rate of body fat may be measured in several ways. Body fat can also be measured by DEXA (dual emission X-ray analysis) in a research setting (and some physician offices), which can be performed on the same equipment used to conduct bone mineral density scans. That is regarded as the best treatment. Inexpensive bio-electrical impedance analysis (BIA) instruments for home use can provide useful information and are available in tools such as a handheld device grasped like a steering wheel, or some home scales. Weighing underwater is another way to measure body fat, and is practiced in some health clubs. The right amounts of body fat appear in the table below. The average American man has a body fat percentage of 24.5 percent, and the average woman has a body fat of 33 percent.

Keeping track of your performance concerning an exercise or physical activity can help you stay motivated for a more extended time. Similarly, the dietary record is also helpful in estimating the daily intake and calories consumed per day. Excluding the habits of using a salt shaker and avoiding high sodium packaged products can help sodium intake in moderation. Diet, as suggested by the dietary approaches to stop hypertension (DASH), is low in sodium, fat, and sugar content and high in fiber, protein, and fresh and organic food products that ultimately improve the overall health of a person. Weight reduction has been proven to reduce the occurrence of other diseases that are associated with high blood pressure. For example, it will prevent the premature stiffening of the arteries and will reduce the risk of stroke or heart attack.

Keto For Women Over 50

Your Tailor-Made Program To Deflate The Belly, Abdominal Fat, And Tone The Muscles. LOSE WEIGHT EASILY WITH THE KETO DIET TO EXPERIENCE A HAPPY MENOPAUSE.

Author: Keli Bay

Introduction: You Can Have A Perfect Body Even At 50

It's not in your brain, women - people don't live in an equivalent world with regards to muscle to fat ratio. Men, with their taller bodies and profound muscle tissues and bones, lay pronounce to snappier digestion. At adolescence, young ladies put on fat, and young men apply on muscle. From breastfeeding to preparation, young ladies have and need more noteworthy fats than men. In this part, we will investigate the advantages and inconveniences of IF and how ladies more than 50 should move toward the eating regimen.

At the point when you quick, your body consumes fat rather than sugar for vitality, which brings about fat misfortune and gives your mind a lift.

Like a car, your body needs fuel to run; Food is that fuel. During digestion, the stomach breaks down the carbohydrates in the sugar that the cells use for energy, to "feed," so to speak. If your cells do not use all the available glucose, eventually, the fat is retained, as you have already guessed. During fasting, your cells go from using glucose as the main source of fuel to consuming fat.

Therefore, fat deposits, mainly triglycerides, are burned for energy. Therefore, research has found that IF can help you lose weight while maintaining muscle mass.

It gives protection from epileptic seizures, Alzheimer's sickness and other neurodegenerative issues.

Exactly when your body uses fat stores for imperativeness, it releases unsaturated fats called ketones into the circulatory framework. Ketones assume a job in weight reduction yet have been appeared to keep up cerebrum work, giving even some protection from epileptic seizures, Alzheimer's malady and other neurodegenerative issues.

For example, a study in older adults with mild cognitive impairment found that an increase in ketones improved memory in just six weeks. Such benefits can occur because ketones secrete brain-derived neurotrophic factor (BDNF), which improves neuronal connections, especially in areas involved in memory and learning.

Studies have shown that if it stimulates the growth of new neurons in the brain.

When you fast, your insulin levels drop, while your human growth hormone and norepinephrine levels rise, which helps you weaken and withstand chronic diseases.

Put simply, we get a torrent of insulin when we eat, while levels drop when we fast. Insulin regulates whether additional glucose from digestion is stored in the body in the form of fat, another reason why IF can contribute to weight loss.

Research shows that IF dramatically lowers insulin and can reduce hyperinsulinemia, as well as improve insulin sensitivity. In animal studies, IF was tested for both diabetes prevention and reversal.

Research also suggests that when insulin is low, and the body registers an increase in transcription factors, which control metabolism-related genes. Finally, this process can change the expression of genes in favor of healthy aging and longevity.

IF also appears to decrease insulin-like growth factors, a genetic marker for diseases such as cancer.

Studies show the arrival of HGH. This is noteworthy on the grounds that, as we become more seasoned, our bodies respond and may bring down the creation of HGH, and this is related to expanded fat tissue and loss of bulk. Exploration of the impact of HGH on body structure proposes that it can assist subjects with getting more fit without losing muscle.

This peak of this neurotransmitter, which you can call it also the stress hormone, contributes to the positive impact of IF on metabolism and helps the body break down fat as a fuel.

Intermittent fasting in what society calls it, interchange day fasting, despite the fact that there is absolutely a few minor departures from this eating regimen. The Journal of Clinical Nutrition executed a glance at nowadays that enlisted 16 hefty guys and females on a 10-week program. On the fasting days, members benefited from food to 25% of their assessed power needs. The remainder of the time, they got healthful directing; notwithstanding, were not, at this point given a particular core value to follow all through this time.

As expected, the participants misplaced weight because of this observe, however, what researchers determined thrilling have been some unique changes. The topics had been all still obese after simply ten weeks, but they'd shown development in cholesterol, LDL-systolic blood pressure, triglycerides, and cholesterol. What made this a thrilling find turned into that most people must lose greater weight than these take a look at participants before seeing the equal changes. It was a captivating find which has spurred an exceptional range of human beings to try fasting.

Intermittent fasting for girls has some useful effects. What makes it especially essential for older girls who are trying to lose weight is that they have a far higher fats proportion in our bodies. When trying to lose weight, the frame, on the whole, burns through carbohydrate stores with the first 6 hours and then begins to burn fats. Women over 50 who are following a healthy food plan and exercise plan may be struggling with stubborn fats, but fasting is a realistic technique to this.

Chapter 28: The Ketogenic Diet: Why It Is Called Ketogenic

People who engage in Keto diet, particularly those aged 50 and older, are said to reap various potential health benefits including:

Improved Physical And Mental Strength

At the point when a person establishes more developed, vitality levels that fall for an assortment of ecological and organic reasons. Disciples to the Keto diet regularly experience a lift in quality and imperativeness. One explanation the event is on the grounds that the body consumes abundance fat, which is combined into vitality thusly.

Metabolism

Maturing individuals regularly experience a more slow digestion than they have encountered in their more youthful days. Long haul keto health food nuts experience expanded blood glucose control, which may improve their metabolic rates.

Protection Against Specific Diseases

Keto dieters over 50 years of age may reduce their risk of developing diseases such as diabetes, mental disorders such as Alzheimer's, various cardiovascular diseases, various types of cancer, Parkinson's disease, non-alcoholic fatty liver disease (NAFLD) and multiple sclerosis.

Good news from the technical description of the ketosis cycle mentioned earlier, reveals the increased energy of the youth as a consequence and because of the use of fat as a source of fuel, the body can go through a phase where signals can be misinterpreted so that the mTOR signal is blocked and a loss of insulin is apparent where aging is stated to be slowed down.

Multiple studies have commonly recognized for years that what cab help you slow your aging process is through caloric restriction and even increasing the lifespan. With the ketogenic diet, it is important to influence anti-aging without increasing calories. The periodic form of fasting used with the keto diet may also impact vascular aging.

The Ketogenic Diet

The Ketogenic Diet follows a simple principle: keep your food consumption low-carb and high-fat. So basically, being on the diet means eating fewer carbohydrates and adding more fats in your daily meals. Do not be confused. When we say "fat" we are not talking about the literal kind that is attached to your body. Fat has gotten a bad reputation nowadays, but "fat" the nutrient is actually very different from the "fat" that makes your clothes fit tight.

Good fats are the kind you get from avocado, nuts, and fish. For example, there are the omega-3 and omega-6 fatty acids that help you lose weight, get better heart health, and have excellent hair and nails.

Naturally, the question that is asked about the Keto Diet is why so many of your friends who are on the Keto Diet seem to be losing so much weight so quickly. The reality is that in the first three to six months on the Keto diet, the body is dropping a tremendous amount of weight because of how the diet is forcing the body to draw energy. Remember how it was said earlier how the body likes to use blood sugar because blood sugar is an easy way to draw energy without using too much energy? Well, what happens when the blood sugar is not in large supply?

This is the essence of weight loss with the Keto Diet. The reality is that weight loss occurs because it takes a lot of calories to burn a single fat cell compared to the calories needed to use blood sugar. The same is true for the protein that is in the body. There is also a psychological element at play here. Carbs can be empty calories and they are really easy to convert into energy – in fact, as you are chewing a piece of bread the body is getting the nutrients from it, whereas if you are eating something that is denser – like meat – then what happens is the digestion occurs in the stomach. It takes much energy to digest a high fat, high protein diet. And – here is the good news – who does not like to have a diet where they can eat things that they love?! This is the great part about the Keto Diet. The high fat and high protein that goes into the diet provides what the body needs in calories to fire up the burning of the fat cells that are critical to losing weight.

When a human fast intermittently or is developed on a keto diet, it is suspected that BHB or Beta-Hydroxybutyrate causes anti-aging results.

Very little in carbs and regularly solid in fats or potentially proteins, ketogenic eats less are utilized effectively for weight reduction during overweight and coronary illness care. Be that as it may, a significant note in the article was that "Results on the effect of such weight control plans on cardiovascular hazard factors are questionable" and "furthermore, these eating regimens are not totally protected and might be related to some unfriendly occasions. More is required than simply investigating this eating routine, points of interest, constructive outcomes, and reactions, especially in matured grown-ups on the Internet. One ought to address their clinical expert about explicit concerns.

Even before we talk about how to do keto – it is important to first consider why this diet works. What happens to your body to make you lose weight?

As you probably know, the body uses food as an energy source. Everything you eat is turned into energy, so that you can get up and do whatever you need to accomplish for the day. The main energy source is sugar so what happens is that you eat something, the body breaks it down into sugar, and the sugar is processed into energy. Typically, the "sugar" is taken directly from the food you eat so if you eat just the right amount of food, then your body is fueled for the whole day. If you eat too much, then the sugar is stored in your body – hence the accumulation of fat.

But what happens if you eat less food? This is where the Ketogenic Diet comes in. You see, the process of creating sugar from food is usually faster if the food happens to be rich in carbohydrates. Bread, rice, grain, pasta – all of these are carbohydrates and they are the easiest food types to turn into energy.

So, the Ketogenic Diet is all about reducing the number of carbohydrates you eat. Does this mean you will not get the kind of energy you need for the day? Of course not! It only means that now, your body must find other possible sources of energy. Do you know where they will be getting that energy? Your stored body fat!

So, here is the situation – you are eating fewer carbohydrates every day. To keep you energetic, the body breaks down the stored fat and turns them into molecules called ketone bodies. The process of turning the fat into ketone bodies is called "Ketosis" and obviously – this is where the name of the Ketogenic Diet comes from. The ketone bodies take the place of glucose in keeping you energetic. If you keep your carbohydrates reduced, the body will keep getting its energy from your body fat.

Sounds Simple, Right?

The Ketogenic Diet is often praised for its simplicity and when you look at it properly, the process is straightforward. The Science behind the effectivity of the diet is also well-documented and has been proven multiple times by different medical fields. For example, an article on Diet Assessment by Harvard provided a lengthy discussion on how the Ketogenic Diet works and why it is so effective for those who choose to use this diet.

But Fat Is the Enemy...Or Is It?

No – fat is NOT the enemy. Unfortunately, years of bad science told us that fat is something you must avoid – but it is actually an extremely helpful thing for weight loss! Even before we move forward with this guide, we will have to discuss exactly what "healthy fats" are, and why they are the good guys. To do this, we need to make a distinction between the different kinds of fat. You have probably heard of them before and it is a little bit confusing at first. We will try to go through them as simply as possible:

Saturated fat. This is the kind you want to avoid. They are also called "solid fat" because each molecule is packed with hydrogen atoms. Simply put, it is the kind of fat that can easily cause a blockage in your body. It can raise cholesterol levels and lead to heart problems or a stroke. Saturated fat is something you can find in meat, dairy products, and other processed food items. Now, you are probably wondering: isn't the Ketogenic Diet packed with saturated fat? The answer is: not necessarily. You will find in the recipes given that the Ketogenic Diet promotes primarily unsaturated fat or healthy fat. While there are many meat recipes on the list, most of these recipes contain healthy fat sources.

Unsaturated Fat. These are the ones dubbed as a healthy fat. They are the kind of fat you find in avocado, nuts, and other ingredients you usually find in Keto-friendly recipes. They are known to lower blood cholesterol and come in two types: polyunsaturated and monounsaturated. Both are good for your body, but the benefits slightly vary, depending on what you are consuming.

Polyunsaturated fat. These are perhaps the best on the list. You know about omega-3 fatty acids, right? They are often suggested for people who have heart problems and are recognized as the "healthy" kind of fat. Well, they fall under the category of polyunsaturated fat and are known for reducing risks of heart disease by as much as 19 percent. This is according to a study titled: Effects on coronary heart diseases of increased poly-unsaturated fat in lieu of saturated fat: systematic assessment & meta-analysis of randomized controlled tests. So where do you get these polyunsaturated fats? You can get them mostly from vegetable and seed oils. These are ingredients you can almost always find in Ketogenic Recipes such as olive oil, coconut oil, and more. If you need more convincing, you should also know that omega-3 fatty acids are a kind of polyunsaturated fats and you will find them in deep sea fish like tuna, herring, and salmon.

Carbohydrates in a regular meal generally make up most of the calories. Also, as it is easier to absorb, the body is inclined to use the carbohydrate as energy. Therefore, the diet's proteins and fats are more likely to be stored.

The body resorts to its stored fat content because of this apparent shortage. It makes a shift from a consumer of carbohydrates to a fat burner. However, in the recently ingested meal, the body does not use the fats, but instead stores them for another round of ketosis.

The body still needs a constant supply of energy during fasting periods-such as during ketosis, between meals and during sleep. You have these times in your normal day, so you need to consume enough fat to use your body as energy. A keto diet's main goal is to mimic the body's hunger state. By restricting and severely reducing the intake of carbohydrates, keto diets deprive the body of its preferred immediate and easily convertible carbohydrates. This situation forces it into a mode of fat burning to produce energy.

Chapter 29: How Long Should It Last?

Many women want to lose weight, but women over the age of 50 are particularly interested in losing weight, boosting their immune system, and having more energy.

If you fit into this group, this phase will address the particular hurdles you may face when doing the Keto diet. For one thing, women in this age range experience slowing metabolisms, making it harder to drop pounds than ever before.

I will cover the tweaks you can make to your Keto diet and lifestyle to accommodate these particular hurdles. I will address any concerns you may have and give you solutions to counteract them.

Women go through menopause sometime between the ages of 45 and 55, and it can be a particularly difficult time. They notice they are putting on weight, and they experience all kinds of unpleasant symptoms such as difficulty sleeping and hot flashes.

But many of these symptoms are temporary. The one that bothers women the most is the one that lasts: weight gain. Women over 50 want to know how they can stave off weight gain and lose the extra pounds they started to put on after menopause.

First of all, I highly recommend intermittent fasting for women in this age group. Intermittent fasting is often paired with Keto for the best possible results in autophagy. Autophagy can be improved through Keto alone, but you don't truly unlock the potential advanced autophagy in your body until you fast between your Ketogenic meals.

The reason I urge you to do intermittent fasting with Keto is that it will help you more with the effects of aging than Keto alone. The autophagy that results from fasting doesn't only help you get better skin, lose weight, and detox your cells—although all these things are worth trying to achieve on their own.

The long-term, anti-aging benefits of intermittent fasting are more important but often ignored. The autophagy that comes from intermittent fasting will help you lower your inflammation, boost your metabolism, enhance your immune system, and more. These are all benefits of autophagy that are backed by scientific research.

Studies show time and time again that fasting works to help women lose weight and improve their health. As a woman over 50, you should consider doing Keto together with fasting.

Scientists are not in agreement about whether menopause itself affects weight. Some say that when women gain weight at this stage in life, it is because of aging alone. They do not believe the hormonal changes from menopause are the reason for the weight gain.

But there is no denying that the lowered estrogen from menopause has some impact on the distribution of fat on the body of a woman over 50. You may have noticed this yourself in your own body: the change in hormones tends to make a woman's fat go from her hips to her waist.

That isn't all, either. Women who go through menopause also report that they have less energy and have a harder time burning fat. It is no wonder women over 50 want to know how to lose weight. It is such a harder feat at this stage in life.

But don't be misled to believe the change in metabolism is all that is going on here. After all, a doctor studying women over 50 found that women's bodies only metabolized 50 calories fewer calories every day. While this is not a negligible figure, it can hardly be blamed for all of the weight gain that is experienced by women at this age.

You are sure to have experienced some of the other factors that play into weight gain for women at this age. Women over 50 report having more cravings, doing less exercise, and losing more muscle.

As you might guess, many of these factors are related. When you aren't exercising as much, you won't retain as much muscle. If you have more cravings for foods you shouldn't eat, you are more likely to eat those foods and gain weight as a result.

Top it all off with the less efficient metabolisms of women over 50, and it is easy to understand why they have a hard time losing weight. Even if menopause itself isn't the reason women experience this, it all adds up to make weight loss seem impossible, if you don't know anything about Keto or fasting.

Take everything you hear them say about weight gain for women over 50 with a grain of salt. All of us know that it is a reality for women who fall into this age range, but no one knows exactly what the reason for it is. But we do know that Keto and fasting both show fantastic results for these women, so that is the information we should really be paying attention to.

Women in this age range can still go wrong when they try Keto and autophagy, so I have some pieces of advice to give you if you count yourself among this group.

The first piece of advice is to make sure you eat enough protein every day. You might be worried about eating too much protein because you are watching calories, and this is a reasonable thing to do. But when you are on Keto, you need protein as a source of energy.

It is always about balance. On the one hand, you need to make up for the energy you won't be getting from carbs. On the other hand, you have to be careful not to eat too many calories.

As usual, follow along with what your body is telling you. If your body tells you that you still need more energy, wait a bit. You can eat more if some time passes and you still feel hungry.

That probably means you need food for energy. But you have to give yourself this waiting period because otherwise, your mind might be trying to trick you into just eating something you are craving when you are not genuinely hungry.

There is a mental component to this change in diet, too. The problem at the center of women not being able to change their diet is not being used to the real feeling of being full.

By the "real" feeling of being full, I am referring to how people feel when they have eaten enough—not too much.

These days, people eat so many carbs that their idea of fullness is the uncomfortable feeling they have when they eat too many carbs. But you can't lose weight if you see fullness this way. You will consistently overstuff yourself, believing you are making yourself full when you are actually gorging yourself.

To remind yourself what fullness actually feels like, get used to eating without overstuffing yourself. Get used to not feeling uncomfortable after eating. It can feel strangely comforting to be overstuffed with carbs, but that is not a feeling we can let ourselves get used to. If we do, we will never be happy with the simple feeling of fullness.

As I keep emphasizing, we can't villainize fat anymore. The real problem is eating too many calories, most of which tend to come from carbs, not fats. However, women over 50, in particular, need to be careful not to eat too many fats when they follow Keto.

Keto isn't a valid excuse for simply eating a ton of fat. You still need to show some constraint as you do in every diet.

Understanding how to balance your fat consumption will take understanding of how fat fits into Keto. With Keto, you want to be what we call fat-adapted.

You already know what this means; it is just another way of saying what happens in Ketosis. Being fat-adapted means, you are burning fat for energy with Ketones instead of burning glucose with carbs.

I tell you this term because you should eat a lot of healthy fats until you go through significant Ketosis—until you are fat-adapted. Once that happens, you should start being more careful with how much fat you are consuming.

One of the sources women over 50 will get fat from is drinks. Even the drinks you make at home like coffee with milk can be a lot higher in fat than you think. It should go without saying that the specialty coffee you get topped with whipped cream is high in fat.

Women over 50 know they have their own hurdles to overcome when they chase the goals of weight loss and improved overall health with Keto. But they can do all they can possibly do by following along with the advice in this phase.

Chapter 30: What to Eat?

Cheese and a Healthy Ketogenic Meal

Definition of Cheese

You probably already know that cheese is a dairy product that is obtained from milk. It consists of casein, a milk protein, and can be produced in several distinct flavors. Cheese is made up of protein and fat and is usually from the milk produced by either sheep, goats, buffaloes, or cows. During the production process of cheese, the milk from these animals is acidified. Rennet, a type of enzyme, is added to the acidified milk leading to coagulation. Calcium, fat, protein, and phosphorus are nutrients present in cheese. Cheese is also known for its ability to last for long periods of time life compared to regular milk.

Types of Cheese

There are numerous known brands of cheese across cultures in the world, and because of this, cheese is classified by; method of making and its length of life, texture, animal milk, place of origin, fat content.

Health Benefits of Using Cheese

As stated earlier, cheese is rich in nutrients such as calcium, fat, and iron, which for you on a Keto diet is essential. Similarly, cheese contains zinc, phosphorus, and vitamins;

some of the essential requirements for the human body. Cheese, a dairy product, could be better positioned to protect your teeth from cavities.

According to research and study, some types of cheese comprises bits of conjugated linoleic acid, which may help your body against obesity and heart diseases. The calcium in cheese is responsible for strengthening your bones. Cheese, through its containment of vitamin B, is essential in maintaining a healthy and glowing youthful skin.

Risks Associated with the Consumption of Cheese

Cheese does not have fiber, and the ingestion of large amounts could lead to constipation. If you are a lactose-intolerant person, the consumption of cheese could be a challenge for you. This is because cheese comprises lactose, which your body might not be able to digest since it lacks the accountable enzymes for breaking it down. Worry not! Some types of cheese, parmesan, are low in lactose, which might be a benefit if you are a lactose intolerant individual. Casein is a milk protein that you may be sensitive to, and even the low lactose cheese may not be suggested for you.

Recommended Cheese for a Healthy Keto Diet

Mozzarella cheese which contains;

5.5g of proteins

86 Calories

1g of carbs

142 mg of calcium

6g fat

Feta cheese which contains;

4g of fat

61 Calories

5g of protein

1g of carbs

59g Calcium

Fruits and Vegetables and a Healthy Ketogenic Meal

What Are Fruits and Vegetables?

Essentially vegetables are plant parts that are eatable by man as food. The parts include stems, seeds, or even flowers. Potatoes and carrots are classified as vegetables since they are edible by human beings. Vegetables are a central part of any meal since they offer vitamins D, B, C, A carbohydrates, and minerals, which are vital for the body in general. Some of the common vegetables worldwide include; potatoes, broccoli, carrots, cabbage (red and green) spinach, legumes, lettuce, onions, and tomatoes.

Fruits are fleshy and frequently the sweet parts of a certain plant that has seeds in them and is edible by man. Human beings across time have depended on fruits as a source of food as well as a way of continuing the growth of plants by replanting the seeds found in the fruits. Most fruits are edible by man in their raw state and may not require any form of cooking before ingesting. Some of the common fruits across cultures in the world include; bananas, oranges, grapes, strawberries, and apples

Fruits and Vegetables That Support the Ketogenic Diet

However, most fruits are high in carbs, and therefore, they are often ignored during a Keto diet plan. However, berries are low in carbs and wealthier in fiber, making them friendly to the Keto diet. Berries (raspberries, strawberries, blackberries, and blueberries) carry antioxidants, which are important in the human body in that they protect you against diseases.

Vegetables are very healthy and are very good for you. If and only if you are on the Keto diet, should you worry about vegetables. As stated in this cook guide, the Keto diet backs a high in fat and low in carb diet plan; you might want to do away with some vegetables that are high in carbs. Carrots and potatoes (sweet potatoes as well as regular potatoes) are high in starch and could possibly interfere with the ketosis process even when ingested in small quantities. Instead, spinach, bell peppers, zucchini, cauliflower, cabbage, broccoli, asparagus, celery, arugula, onion, olives, and pumpkins are all Keto-friendly and thus recommended for your usage.

Why the Ketogenic Fruit and Vegetable Bread?

Any diet rich in fruits and vegetables, the Ketogenic fruit and vegetable bread included, is beneficial to you in that it lowers your chances of suffering from heart diseases. The dietary fiber contained in vegetables is important because it is responsible for the lowering of your body's blood cholesterol levels and reduce your risk of heart diseases. This bread offers you a chance to reduce your chances of developing cardiovascular diseases

This bread also gives you a chance to minimize your chances of coming into contact with cancer. You already know that cancer is deadly, and the mere fact that the bread offers you a shield against cancer should be reason enough for you to bake and consume. The Keto fruit and vegetable bread also lowers your chances of developing prostate cancer if you are a man.

The Keto fruit and vegetable bread also lowers your risk of contracting diabetes.

The fiber in these fruits and vegetable bread is essential in ensuring your digestive system is smooth.

Types of Sweeteners That Support the Keto Diet

As stated earlier in thiscook guidee, ketogenic diets advocate for cutting back in high carbs foods, for example, processed snacks. This is important for you if you want your body to reach the ketosis stage and burn fat instead of carbs to produce energy for your body. Ketosis is also a result of low sugar consumption, which could pose a challenge if you want to sweeten your bread. Lucky for you, there are actually low carb sweeteners that support the Keto diet.

Xylitol - This is a type of sugar alcohol that is usually found in candies, sugar-free gum as well as mints. You may use this sweetener for baking, but you would need more liquids because it tends to increase dryness in the dough as a result of its moisture-absorbent nature. The carbs in this sweetener do not raise your blood sugar levels or insulin levels, unlike the regular sugar.

Note: Xylitol, when used in high amounts, may cause digestive issues; thus, you should be careful with the amounts you use.

Sucralose - this sweetener passes through your body undigested simply because it is a non-metabolized artificial sweetener that has no carbs or calories, making it popular on the markets since it lacks the bitter test common in many artificial sweeteners.

Stevia – This is a natural sweetener that contains very little amount of carbs or calories. It is from the stevia rebaudiana plant, and unlike the regular sugar, stevia may be useful in lowering blood sugar levels. This sweetener can be found in both the liquids and the powder states, and you could use it to sweeten your food or drinks.

Note: Stevia is much sweeter than regular sugar; thus, you should be careful with the amounts you desire in either your food or drinks or even when using it in a recipe.

Monk fruit sweetener – It is a natural sweetener, and it contains no calories as well as no carbs, which is an essential element in the maintenance of a ketogenic diet. This sweetener is extracted from a plant in China called the monk fruit. The sweetness of this natural sweetener is a result of the natural compounds and sugars, which are antioxidants. This sweetener is essential for regulating blood sugar levels in your body.

Note: You could decide to use the monk fruit sweetener in the place of regular sugar, but you should be in a position to reduce the amount of the sweetener in half in order to achieve the required results.

Why Sweeteners Instead of Regular Sugar?

You might probably be asking yourself this very question. Well, the answer is simple. Sweeteners, like the regular sugar, provide a sweet test during consumption, but what sweeteners have over regular sugar is the ability to not increase the body's blood sugar levels. Extensive conduction of research studies has proven that sweeteners are safe for consumption on a daily basis. For instance, if you are suffering from diabetes, the use of sweetness is useful to you because you do not have to worry about your body's blood sugar levels when you are out enjoying your meals with family and friends.

On a normal diet, human beings consume up to 50% to 55% of carbohydrates. That is more than half the percentage of the whole meal. Proteins take up about 25% of the remaining meal, while fats take up the remaining 20%. This is contrary to the Ketogenic diet, which constitutes about 75% of fats, 20% of protein, and only 5% of carbohydrates. For instance, if you weigh 160 pounds and you are averagely active, then your body would require approximately 30 grams of carbohydrates, 90 grams of protein, and 200 grams of fats for a single day while on the Ketogenic diet.

Cholesterol; is an organic molecule and is important in the structure of the cell membranes. The normal cholesterol levels in an adult are less than 200 mg/dl (milligrams per deciliter). The Ketogenic diet has been reported to regulate the cholesterol levels of some people who adopted the diet. The diet decreases the levels of triglycerides, blood sugar as well as LDL cholesterol.

Protein; it is recommended to ingest between 0.6 – 1.0 grams of protein per pound in the weight of your body (1.6 – 2.0 grams per kilogram). Note that consuming protein in large amounts could get your body out of ketosis.

Fat; the levels of calories originating from fats will depend on how low your consumption of carbohydrates is, and this is probably between 55 – 80%. You could consume;

1,600 calories for about 85 – 130 grams of fat in a day

2,000 calories for about 115 – 170 grams of fat in a day

2,500 calories for about 140 – 210 grams of fat in a day

Carbohydrates; it should be noted that there is no set limit for carbs in a Ketogenic diet. However, anything below 100 grams is considered low carb. You could achieve ketosis is you ate unprocessed real foods.

Sugar; Ketogenic diet ensures you abstain from all foods with carbs, including refined sugar. This means sugar should be limited as low as possible to ensure your body gets into nutritional ketosis.

Grain and dairy; grains and dairy products are rich in carbs, which is against the Ketogenic diet, meaning you have to minimize your consumption to fit in the daily less than 100 grams of carbs.

Chapter 31: How Ketogenic Metabolism Works

Ketosis is a standard metabolic procedure that offers various wellbeing favorable circumstances.

During ketosis, your body changes over fat into mixes known as ketones and begins to utilize them as its essential wellspring of vitality.

Studies have found that consumes fewer calories that energize ketosis are very valuable for weight reduction owing to some degree to hunger suppressant impacts.

Rising examination shows that ketosis may likewise be valuable for, among different conditions, type 2 diabetes and neurological issue.

That being stated, accomplishing ketosis can set aside some effort to work and plan. It's not as simple as cutting carbs.

Here are some productive tips for getting into ketosis.

Reduce Your Carb Consumption

Expending a low carb diet is by a wide margin the most critical factor in achieving ketosis.

Typically, your phones use glucose or sugar as their essential fuel source. In any case, the majority of your cells can likewise utilize different wellsprings of vitality. This includes unsaturated fats, just as ketones, which are otherwise called ketones.

Your body stores glucose in the liver and muscles as glycogen.

At the point when the utilization of starches is extremely little, the glycogen stores decline and the hormone insulin focuses decline. This empowers unsaturated fats to be discharged from your muscle versus fat's shops.

Your liver changes a bit of these unsaturated fats to ketone, acetoacetate and beta-hydroxybutyrate. These ketones can be used as fuel for parts of the cerebrum.

The proportion of carb obstruction required to cause ketosis is somewhat individualized. A couple of individuals need to bind net carbs (complete carbs short fiber) to 20 grams for consistently, while others can accomplish ketosis by eating twice so a great deal or more.

Subsequently, the Atkins diet confirms that carbs should be confined to 20 or fewer grams for consistently for around fourteen days to ensure that ketosis is cultivated.

After this stage, modest quantities of carbs can be familiar with your eating routine a little bit at a time, as long as ketosis is ensured.In a one-week research, people with type 2 diabetes who had limited carb utilization to 21 grams or less every day experienced day by day urinary ketone discharge rates that were multiple times more noteworthy than their standard fixations.

In another exploration, grown-ups with type 2 diabetes were allowed 20–50 grams of edible carbs every day, in light of the number of grams that allowed blood ketone focuses on being kept up inside the objective scope of 0.5–3.0 mmol/L.

These carb and ketone ranges are prescribed for people who need to get ketosis to energize weight reduction, control glucose fixations or lessening hazard factors for coronary illness.

Helpful ketogenic abstains from food utilized for epilepsy or exploratory disease treatment, then again, regularly limit carbs to under 5 percent of calories or under 15 grams for each day to additionally build ketone levels.

Nonetheless, any individual who utilizes an eating regimen for restorative reasons should just do as such under the direction of a clinical expert.

Restricting your starch utilization to 20–50 net grams for every day lessens glucose and insulin fixations, prompting the arrival of putting away unsaturated fats that your liver proselytes to ketones.

Incorporate Coconut Oil In Your Diet

The utilization of coconut oil can help you to get into ketosis.

It incorporates fats called medium-chain triglycerides (MCTs).

In contrast to most fats, MCTs are immediately ingested and taken directly to the liver, where they can be utilized in a split second for vitality or changed to ketones.

As a general rule, it has been proposed that the utilization of coconut oil might be perhaps the most ideal approach to help ketone focuses on people with Alzheimer's ailment and different sensory system diseases.

Despite the fact that coconut oil incorporates four sorts of MCTs, half of its fat is gotten from the sort known as lauric corrosive.

A few examinations propose that fat sources with a more noteworthy extent of lauric corrosive may produce a progressively consistent measure of ketosis. This is on the grounds that it is more continuously used than different MCTs.

MCTs have been utilized to cause ketosis in epileptic children without restricting carbs as definitely as the exemplary ketogenic diet.

In actuality, a few preliminaries have found that a high-MCT diet including 20 percent of starch calories creates impacts tantamount to the great ketogenic diet, which offers under 5 percent of sugar calories.

While adding coconut oil to your eating routine, it's a smart thought to do so gradually to limit stomach related reactions, for example, stomach squeezing or loose bowels.

Start with one teaspoon daily and work up to a few tablespoons every day for seven days. You can find coconut oil in your neighborhood supermarket or get it on the web.

Devouring coconut oil offers your body with MCTs that are quickly retained and changed into ketone bodies by your liver.

Enhance Your Physical Activity

An expanding measure of examination has demonstrated that ketosis can be helpful for certain sorts of athletic execution, including continuance work out.

What's more, being progressively dynamic may help you get into ketosis.

At the point when you practice, your body will be drained from its glycogen shops. Typically, these are renewed when you expend carbs that are separated into glucose and afterward changed to glycogen.

In any case, if the utilization of sugar is limited, the glycogen shops remain little. In response, your liver improves the yield of ketones, which can be utilized as an elective wellspring of vitality for your body.

One examination found that activity improves the rate at which ketones are produced at low blood ketone levels. Be that as it may, when blood ketones are raised, they don't increment with practice and may viably diminish for a short timeframe.

Also, it has been demonstrated that turning out to be in a fasted state is driving up ketone focuses.

In a little examination, nine old females performed either preceding or after a supper. Their blood ketone focuses were 137–314 percent more prominent when utilized before a supper than when utilized after a dinner.

Remember that despite the fact that activity rises ketone yield, it might take one to about a month for your body to acclimate to the utilization of ketones and unsaturated fats as principle energizes. Physical execution might be diminished immediately during this second.

Taking part in physical activity may support ketone fixations during carb restriction. This effect can be improved by working in a quick paced state.

Ramp Up Your Healthy Fat Intake

A lot of good fat can expand your ketone focuses and assist you with accomplishing ketosis.

Indeed, an exceptionally low-carb ketogenic diet limits carbs as well as high in fat.

Ketogenic eats less carbs for weight reduction, metabolic wellbeing and exercise proficiency by and large give between 60-80 percent of fat calories.

The exemplary ketogenic diet utilized for epilepsy is significantly more noteworthy in fat, with commonly 85–90 percent of calories in fat.

Be that as it may, incredibly raised fat utilization doesn't really bring about more prominent ketone focuses.

A three-week exploration of 11 sound individuals differentiated the effects of fasting with particular amounts of fat utilization on ketone centralizations of relaxing.

In general, ketone focuses have been found to be tantamount in people who expend 79% or 90% of fat calories.

Additionally, on the grounds that fat makes up such a major extent of the ketogenic diet, it is fundamental to pick top notch sources.

Extraordinary fats consolidate olive oil, avocado oil, coconut oil, spread, oil and sulfur. Moreover, there are various strong, high-fat sustenances that are in like manner little in carbs.

Nevertheless, if your goal is weight decrease, it's fundamental to guarantee you don't exhaust such countless calories inside and out, as this can make your weight decrease delayed down.

Exhausting on any occasion 60 percent of fat calories will help increase your ketone centers. Pick the extent of sound fats from both animal and plant sources.

Try A Fat Fast Or Short Fast

The other method to get into ketosis is to abandon eating for a couple of hours.

Actually, numerous people have gentle ketosis among lunch and breakfast.

Youngsters with epilepsy now and then quick for 24–48 hours before they start a ketogenic diet. This is accomplished to get into ketosis quickly with the goal that seizures can be diminished all the more quickly.

Irregular fasting, a wholesome technique including intermittent momentary fasting, may likewise cause ketosis.

Likewise, "fat fasting" is another ketone-boosting system that mirrors the effects of fasting.

It incorporates expending around 1,000 calories every day, 85–90 percent of which originate from fat. This blend of low calories and an extremely raised utilization of fat can help you accomplish ketosis quickly.

A 1965 exploration uncovered a significant loss of fat in overweight patients who followed a speedy fat. Be that as it may, different researchers have called attention to that these discoveries seem to have been incredibly misrepresented.

Since fat is so little in protein and calories, a limit of three to five days ought to be followed to evade an inordinate loss of bulk. It might likewise be difficult to adhere to for in excess of a couple of days.

Fasting, irregular fasting and "fat fasting" would all be able to help you get into ketosis relatively quickly.

Maintaining Adequate Protein Intake

Showing up at ketosis needs a protein use that is fitting anyway not over the top.

The commendable ketogenic diet used in epilepsy patients is obliged to increasing ketone centers in both carbs and proteins.

A comparative eating routine may in like manner be important to infection patients as it would restrain tumor improvement.

In any case, it's definitely not a not too bad practice for the vast majority to decrease proteins to enable ketone to yield.

In any case, it is basic to eat up enough protein to effortlessly the liver with amino acids that can be used for gluconeogenesis, which means' new glucose.' In this strategy, your liver offers glucose to the couple of cells and organs in your body that can't use ketones as fuel.

Chapter 32: The Side Effects Of The Ketogenic Diet

The diet can cause a few side effects, including:

Induction Flu: Symptoms include confusion, brain fog, irritability, lethargy, and nausea. These symptoms are common during the first week of the diet.

The cure: consume salt and water. You can cure all these symptoms by getting enough water and salt into your system. Drinking broth daily is a better option.

Leg Cramps: Leg cramps are painful.

The cure: get enough salt and drink plenty of fluids. Taking magnesium supplements is also a good idea. Take three slow-release magnesium tablets daily for the first three weeks.

Constipation: Constipation is another side effect of the diet.

The cure: Getting enough salt and water. Also, include more fiber in your diet, such as fruits and vegetables.

Bad Breath: Bad breath is another unpleasant problem that may arise.

The cure:

Eat more carbohydrates.

Get enough salt and drink enough fluids

Maintain good oral hygiene.

Heart palpitations

The cure: getting enough fluid is the easiest solution

Generally, you can eliminate all the Keto side effects by:

Drinking more water

Increasing salt intake

Eating enough fat

Myths and Misconceptions Concerning the Ketogenic Diet

As one of its side effects, the formation of what is known as ketones is the breaking down of body fat into fatty acids. These acidic fat metabolism by-products tend to increase the level of acidity of the body when they accumulate in the bloodstream and may degenerate into certain conditions of health.

The use of ketogenic diets is one way that ketones can accumulate in the bloodstream. Ketogenic diets such as the famous Atkins Diet are of the view that carbohydrates are the main cause of weight gain and are designed to limit the amount of carbohydrates eaten every day throughout their diets.

Normally, carbohydrates are digested to generate fructose, which is called the body's favorite form of food as it is a quick burning fuel. While the body can metabolize muscle and liver glycogen (a combination of glucose and water) as well as body fat deposits to generate energy, it tends to receive it from high glycemic carbohydrates.

The initial phase of a ketogenic diet usually involves an acute glucose deprivation designed to force the body to exhaust its own available glucose to a significantly lower level that ultimately forces it to switch to burning its fat deposits for energy.

The rate of lipolysis (breakdown of body fat) increases dramatically at this stage of a ketogenic diet to push the body into a state known as ketosis to meet its energy requirements. Ketosis is a condition in which the rate of formation of ketone bodies (by-products of decomposition of fat into fatty acids) is faster than the rate at which the body tissues oxidize them.

Under normal conditions, ketone bodies are easily oxidized to water and carbon dioxide, but their oxidation is very complicated due to increased aggregation during ketosis. The enhanced concentration of ketones in the bloodstream, though, normally leads to increased body acidity causing the body to continue to use water reserves from its cells to flush out the excess ketones.

Therefore, ketogenic diets are designed to achieve two very important weight loss goals: reducing the production of insulin due to the resulting low blood sugar levels; and also the ketosis state which increases the lipolysis rate (fat breakdown). The addition of these two causes allows the use of a ketogenic diet a very successful way to achieve an accelerated loss of weight.

Sadly, the state of elevated ketone aggregation in the skin has been somewhat inconsistent. This is due in part to the fact that many people fail to realize that apart from the ketosis effect of ketogenic diets, another physiological condition may also cause increased accumulation of ketone.

Including ketosis, the other disorder that can induce an elevated concentration of ketones is ketoacidosis. While there is no doubt that both conditions result in increased ketone accumulation and therefore body acidity, the precipitating conditions are very different, however.

Ketoacidosis (also known as Diabetic Ketoacidosis-DKA) is a serious condition in which ketone bodies accumulate in Type I bloodstream diabetics due to the body's inability to produce enough insulin. An increase in counter-regulatory hormones aggravates this condition.

Insulin deficiency in a diabetic contributes to the hyperglycemia-an excessive rise of blood sugar levels that can be as much as four times the bloodstream's usual amount of sugar. When an excessive increase in blood sugar levels happens in a normal individual, the glomeruli of the kidneys remove more insulin than the kidney tubules can reabsorb, resulting in glucose excretion in the urine.

Hyperglycemia is not that dangerous in and of itself, but the side effects can be life-threatening as it usually results in glycosuria (presence of sugar in the urine), excessive urination, and dehydration. Glucose intake of urine is usually associated with exhaustion, nausea, weight loss, and increased appetite.

Continued glucose excretion from the urine and dehydration makes the body seriously hungry for energy. To keep the situation under control, the body can, on the one side, begin to excrete glucose in the urine which triggers a more severe condition, the Hyperosmolar Hyperglycemia Syndrome (HHS), which in people with this condition has a reported mortality rate of around 15%.

On the other hand, as a way to produce more energy to control the situation, the body can begin to break down more triglycerides (stored body fat). Furthermore, this decreased lipolysis (the removal of fatty acids and ketones from fat cells, muscle tissues, and the liver) induces an elevated concentration of ketones (fat degradation by-products) in the urine and the bloodstream to increase blood acidity. What is known as Diabetic Ketoacidosis-DKA is the combination of hyperglycemia and acidosis (abnormal increase in blood acidity).

Thus, while in all cases there is actually a high volume of residual ketones, there is an increased level of blood sugar in the ketoacidosis system. Actually, ketoacidosis can degenerate into hyperventilation, resulting in a subsequent impairment of functions of the central nervous system that can lead to coma and death.

Therefore, it must be stressed that dietitians who use ketogenic diets will ensure that they drink plenty of water to mitigate the elevated acidity rate of the body induced by the release of ketones. This also allows the stored ketones to wash out and preserve a healthy hydration condition.

To sum up, although ketosis is induced by reduced levels of blood sugar, ketoacidosis is caused by increased levels of blood sugar. Although there may be ketone accumulation in both conditions in the bloodstream and urine, their causes are separate poles, however.

Mistake Made on the Keto Diet and How to Overcome Them.

The most common mistakes revolve around food choices. It is important to maintain correct ratios of fats to proteins. The diet program is subject to failure, and poor health may result in failing to maintain the proper amount of fat. The ketogenic diet is based on using fat to burn as fuel in the body. As a result, the body needs fat to burn. Of course, these need to be good fats that promote increases in HDL cholesterol. This will provide good fuel for the body.

It is important to eat the right fats. Margarine, vegetable oil, canola oil, trans fats, and other light non-viscous plant oils and unhealthy fats should be eliminated from the diet. The fat consumed should be high quality like butter from grass-fed animals, olive oil, monounsaturated oils such as from avocados and coconuts. These are oils and fats are the best options for food and keto. The quality of the fat is important so that it is easily processed and converted to fuel.

Be sure to drink adequate amounts of water when you're on the keto diet. Water will help prevent some of the adverse side effects of the keto diet. It can help with constipation and also help dilute ketones, and acids subject accumulate in the bloodstream. Water is an instrumental factor in avoiding additional weight gain from retention and bloating. You will feel better drinking plenty of water.

Failing to drink adequate amounts of water is a common and unhealthy mistake made by ketogenic dieters. Especially at the beginning of the diet, urination will be frequent. The water needs to be replaced, and you may need to replace electrolytes as well. Make sure to feed your body appropriate nutrients.

When you embark on the keto diet, you may find that you eliminate many processed foods from your diet. These foods use salt as a preservative. Because of this, you will need to replace the salt in your system that you will lose as you drink more water and urinate more frequently. This will help you avoid keto flu or reduce the symptoms of the keto flu.

One of the main mistakes people make on the keto diet is eating too many calories.

There is a myth that you can eat whatever you like on the keto diet as long as it is low or no carb and/ or high in fat. General life principles are still in effect. If you consume more calories than you burn, you'll gain weight. It is important to maintain vigilance in the number of calories consumed and be sure to eat quality foods containing whole grains and fiber. Though there is room in the diet for keto-friendly snacks, try to avoid processed snacks, which may have more carbohydrates than expected. It is important to assess all processed food labels to know the nutritional value of the food you consume.

Chapter 33: The Solution To Your Weight Problems

Routines are very important on this diet, and it's something that will help you stay healthy. As such, in this phase, we are going to be giving you tips and tricks to make this diet work better for you and help you get an idea of routines that you can put in place for yourself.

Tip number one that is so important is DRINK WATER! This is absolutely vital for any diet that you're on, and you need it if not on one as well. However, this vital tip is crucial on a keto diet because when you are eating fewer carbs, you are storing less water, meaning that you are going to get dehydrated very easily. You should aim for more than the daily amount of water however, remember that drinking too much water can be fatal as your kidneys can only handle so much as once. While this has mostly happened to soldiers in the military, it does happen to dieters as well, so it is something to be aware of.

Along with that same tip is to keep your electrolytes. You have three major electrolytes in your body. When you are on a keto diet, your body is reducing the amount of water that you store. It can be flushing out the electrolytes that your body needs as well, and this can make you sick. Some of the ways that you can fight this are by either salting your food or drinking bone broth. You can also eat pickled vegetables.

Eat when you're hungry instead of snacking or eating constantly. This is also going to help, and when you focus on natural foods and health foods, this will help you even more. Eating processed foods is the worst thing you can do for fighting cravings, so you should really get into the routine of trying to eat whole foods instead.

Another routine that you can get into is setting a note somewhere that you can see it that will remind you of why you're doing this in the first place and why it's important to you. Dieting is hard, and you will have moments of weakness where you're wondering why you are doing this. Having a reminder will help you feel better, and it can really help with your perspective.

Tracking progress is something that straddles the fence. A Lot of people say that this helps a lot of people and you can celebrate your wins, however, as everyone is different and they have different goals, progress can be slower in some than others. This can cause others to be frustrated and sad, as well as wanting to give up. One of the most important things to remember is that while progress takes time, and you shouldn't get discouraged if you don't see results right away. With most diets, it takes at least a month to see any results. So don't get discouraged and keep trying if your body is saying that you can. If you can't, then you will need to talk to your doctor and see if something else is for you.

You should make it a daily routine to try and lower your stress. Stress will not allow you to get into ketosis, which is that state that keto wants to put you in. The reason for this being that stress increases the hormone known as cortisol in your blood, and it will prevent your body from being able to burn fats for energy. This is because your body has too much sugar in your blood. If you're going through a really high period of stress right now in your life, then this diet is not a great idea. Some great ideas for this would be getting into the habit or routine of taking the time to do something relaxing, such as walking and making sure that you're getting enough sleep, leads to another routine that you need to do.

You need to get enough sleep. This is so important not just for your diet but also for your mind and body as well. Poor sleep also raises those stress hormones that can cause issues for you, so you need to get into the routine of getting seven hours of sleep at night on the minimum and nine hours if you can. If you're getting less than this, you need to change the routine you have in place right now and make sure that you establish a new routine where you are getting more sleep. As a result, your health and diet will be better.

Another routine that you need to get into is to give up diet soda and sugar substitutes. This is going to help you with your diet as well because diet soda can actually increase your sugar levels to a bad amount, and most diet sodas contain aspartame. This can be a carcinogen, so it's actually quite dangerous. Another downside is that using these sugar substitutes just makes you want more sugar . Instead, you need to get into the habit of drinking water or sparkling water if you like the carbonation.

Staying consistent is another routine that you need to get yourself into. No matter what you are choosing to do, make sure it's something that you can actually do. Try a routine for a couple of weeks and make serious notes of mental and physical problems that you're going through as well as any emotional issues that come your way. Make changes as necessary until you find something that works well for you and that you can stick to it. Remember that you need to give yourself time to get used to this and time to get used to changes before you give up on them.

Be honest with yourself, as well. This is another big tip for this diet. If you're not honest with yourself, this isn't going to work. Another reason that you need to be honest with yourself is if something isn't working you need to be able to understand that and change it. Are you giving yourself enough time to make changes? Are you pushing too hard? If so, you need to understand what is going on with yourself and how you need to deal with the changes that you're going through. Remember not to get upset or frustrated. This diet takes time, and you need to be able to be a little more patient to make this work effectively.

Getting into the routine of cooking for yourself is also going to help you so much on this diet. Eating out is fun, but honestly, on this diet, it can be hard to eat out. It is possible to do so with a little bit of special ordering and creativity, but you can avoid all the trouble by simply cooking for yourself. It saves time, and it saves a lot of cash.

This another topic falls into both the tip and routine category. Get into the habit of cleaning your kitchen. It's very hard to stick to a diet if your kitchen is dirty and full of junk food. Clear out the junk (donate it if you can, even though it's junk, there are tons of hungry people that would appreciate it) and replace all of the bad food with healthy keto food instead. Many people grab the carbs like crazy because they haven't cleared out their cabinets, and it's everywhere they look. Remember, with this diet, no soda, pasta, bread, candy, and things of that nature. Replacing your food with healthy food and making a regular routine of cleaning your kitchen and keeping the bad food out is going to help you be more successful with your diet, which is what you want here.

Getting into the routine of having snacks on hand is a good idea as well. This keeps you from giving into temptation while you're out, and you can avoid reaching for that junk food. You can make sure that they are healthy, and you will be sticking to your high-intensity diet, which is what you want. There are many different keto snacks that you can use for yourself and to eat. We will have a list of recipes in the following phases to help this as well.

A good tip would be to use keto sticks or a glucose meter. This will give you feedback on whether your users do this diet right. The best option here is a glucose meter. It's expensive, but it's the most accurate. Be aware that if you use ketostix, they are cheaper, but the downside is that they are not accurate enough to help you. A perfect example is that they have a habit of telling people their ketone count is low when they are actually the opposite.

Try not to overeat as this will throw you out of where you need to be. Get into the routine of paying attention to what you're eating and how much. If this is something that you're struggling with, try investing in a food scale. You will be able to see exactly what it is your eating and make sure that your understanding your portions and making sure you stay in ketosis.

Another tip is to make sure that you're improving your gut health. This is so important. Your gut is pretty much linked to every other system in your body, so make sure that this something that you want to take seriously. When you have healthy gut flora, your body's hormones, along with your insulin sensitivity and metabolic flexibility will all be more efficient. When your flexibility is functioning at an optimal level, your body is able to adapt to your diet easier. If it's not, then it will convert the fat your trying to use for energy into body fat.

Batch cooking or meal prepping is another routine that is a good thing to get into. This is an especially good routine for on the go women. When you cook in batches, you are able to make sure that you have meals that are ready to go, and you don't have to cook every single day, and you can save a lot of time as well. You will also be making your environment better for your diet because you're supporting your goals instead of working against them.

The last tip is to mention exercise again. Getting into the routine of exercising can boost your ketone levels, and it can help you with your issues on transitioning to keto. Exercises also use different types of energy for your fuel that you need. When your body gets rid of the glycogen storages, it needs other forms of energy, and it will turn into that energy that you need. Just remember to avoid exercises that are going to hurt you. Stay in the smaller exercises and lower intensity.

Following these tips and getting into these routines is going to help you stay on track and make sure that your diet will go as smoothly as it possibly can.

Chapter 34: 7-Day Food Program

Day	Breakfast	Snack	Lunch	Snack	Dinner
1	Scrambled eggs with cheddar cheese, spinach, and sundried tomatoes	Sunflower seeds and mixed nuts	Cauliflower soup with bacon or tofu	Turkey and cucumber roll-ups and celery sticks with guacamole	Garlic and herb shrimp in butter sauce with zucchini noodles

What Do I Eat At Work: Spinach salad with grilled salmon and Melted Cheese

See recipes for lunch and dinner on the following topics.

Day	Breakfast	Snack	Lunch	Snack	Dinner
2	Fried eggs with sautéed greens and pumpkin seeds	Mixed berries and Macadamia nuts	Chicken salad with cucumber, avocado, tomato, onion, and almonds	Almond milk and chia seed smoothie and berries	Beef stew with mushrooms and onions

What Do I Eat At Work: Tuna salad stuffed in tomatoes

See recipes for lunch and dinner on the following topics.

Day	Breakfast	Snack	Lunch	Snack	Dinner
3	Almond milk smoothie containing nut butter, spinach, chia seeds, and protein powder	Greek yogurt accompanied with crushed pecans and an almond milk smoothie with greens and protein powder	Chicken tenders served on a bed of greens with cucumbers and goat cheese	Mixed nuts and sliced cheese with olives and bell peppers	Grilled shrimp topped with lemon and served with broccoli

What Do I Eat At Work: Super-Fast Keto Sandwiches

See recipes for lunch and dinner on the following topics

Day	Breakfast	Snack	Lunch	Snack	Dinner
4	Omelette with mushrooms, bell peppers, and broccoli	Hard-boiled eggs and sliced cheese with sliced bell peppers	Avocado and egg salad served in lettuce cups	Mixed nuts and sliced cheese with olives and bell peppers	Cajun chicken breast with cauliflower rice and Brussels sprouts

What Do I Eat At Work: Slow Cooker Chili with Braised Beef

See recipes for lunch and dinner on the following topics.

Day	Breakfast	Snack	Lunch	Snack	Dinner
5	Fried eggs with bacon and a side of leafy greens	Walnuts with mixed berries and celery dipped in almond butter	Burger in a lettuce bun, accompanied with avocado and served with a side salad	Celery sticks dipped in almond butter and a handful of mixed berries and nuts	Baked tofu with cauliflower rice, broccoli, bell peppers, and a Thai peanut butter sauce

What Do I Eat At Work: Keto Wraps With Cream Cheese And Salmon

See recipes for lunch and dinner on the following topics.

Day	Breakfast	Snack	Lunch	Snack	Dinner
6	Baked eggs served in avocado halves	Kale chips and sugar-free jerky (turkey or beef)	Poached salmon and avocado rolls wrapped in seaweed	Kale chips and sliced cheese and olives	Grilled beef kebabs with peppers and broccoli

What Do I Eat At Work: Keto Croque Monsieur

See recipes for lunch and dinner on the following topics.

Day	Breakfast	Snack	Lunch	Snack	Dinner
7	Scrambled eggs with veggies and salsa	Dried seaweed and cheese slices	Tuna salad made with mayo, served in avocado halves	Sugar-free turkey jerky and an egg and vegetable muffin	Trout broiled with butter and sautéed bok choy

What Do I Eat At Work: Carpaccio

See recipes for lunch and dinner on the following topics.

Chapter 35: Lunch Recipes from the 7-Day Meal Plan

Day 1 - Cauliflower Soup With Bacon Or Tofu

Preparation Time: 20 minutes

Cooking Time: 60 minutes

Serves: 8

Ingredients:

1 medium head cauliflower, broken into florets

2 Tbsp extra virgin olive oil, divided

2 carrots, trimmed and diced

3 celery stalks, trimmed and diced

2 shallots, trimmed and diced

3 garlic cloves, minced

1 lb. silken tofu

3 Tbsp Kikkoman Traditionally Brewed Soy Sauce

8 cups low-sodium chicken or vegetable broth

For topping (optional):

Chives, sliced

Bacon, cooked and crumbled

Directions:

Preheat broiler to 425.

Line a preparing sheet with tinfoil.

Spot cauliflower florets onto the preparing sheet and sprinkle with 1 Tbsp olive oil.

Broil cauliflower for around 40 minutes, flipping part of the way through cooking time, or until brilliant earthy colored and delicate. Expel from broiler.

In the interim, in an enormous soup pot, heat staying 1 Tbsp olive oil over medium warmth.

Include carrots, celery and shallots.

Saute for around 5 minutes, mixing regularly, until vegetables perspire and relax however not earthy colored.

Include garlic and saute one more moment.

Include tofu, separating it in the pot.

Include soy sauce and stock.

Bring to a stew.

When cauliflower is done simmered, add cauliflower to the pot.

Heat to the point of boiling, at that point diminish to a stew for 5-10 minutes.

Expel pot from heat.

Carefully mix soup, utilizing a submersion blender, until smooth.

Spoon soup into bowls and top with chives and disintegrated bacon.

Present with a warm dried up entire baguette roll.

Nutrition:

Calories per serving: 541

Carbohydrates: 4g

Protein: 34g

Fat: 41g

Sugar: 0.1g

Sodium: 164mg

Fiber: 1.2g

Day 2 - Chicken Salad With Cucumber, Avocado, Tomato, Onion, And Almonds

Preparation Time: 15 minutes

Cooking Time: 15 minutes

Serves: 6

Ingredients:

1 Rotisserie chicken deboned and shredded (skin on or off)

1 large English (or continental) cucumber, halved lengthways and sliced into 1/4-inch thick slices

4-5 large Roma tomatoes sliced or chopped

1/4 red onion thinly sliced

2 avocados peeled, pitted and diced

1/2 cup flat leaf parsley chopped*

3 tablespoons olive oil

2-3 tablespoons lemon juice (or the juice of 2 limes)

Salt and pepper to taste

Directions:

Mix together shredded chicken, cucumbers, tomatoes, onion, avocados, and chopped parsley in a large salad bowl.

Drizzle with the olive oil and lemon juice (or lime juice), and season with salt and pepper. Toss gently to mix all of the flavors through.

Nutrition:

Calories per serving: 541

Carbohydrates: 10g

Protein: 40g

Fat: 37g

Sugar: 3g

Sodium: 123mg

Fiber: 6g

Day 3 - Chicken Tenders Served On A Bed Of Greens With Cucumbers And Goat Cheese

Preparation Time: 15 minutes

Cooking Time: 10 minutes

Serves: 6

Ingredients:

boneless skinless chicken

milk

lemon juice

sugar

cornstarch

pepper

breadcrumbs

regular breadcrumbs

all-purpose flour

onion powder

salt or garlic salt

pepper

shortening or oil, for frying

Romaine Lettuce

Cucumber

Goat cheese

Directions:

Quick marinade to tenderize and flavor chicken.

Heat oil for fried chicken tenders

Coat the chicken with simple breading

Fry the coated chicken tenders until golden brown for 10 minutes

On a plate, add rinsed lettuce and chopped cucumber thinly sliced on a half round cut seeds off.

Served with goat cheese on top. Enjoy!

Nutrition:

Calories per serving: 548

Carbohydrates: 3g

Protein: 52g

Fat: 36g

Sugar: 0.1g

Sodium: 175mg

Fiber: 2g

Day 4 - Avocado And Egg Salad Served In Lettuce Cups

Preparation Time: 15 minutes

Cooking Time: 15 minutes

Serves: 2

Ingredients:

1 ripe avocado

1 Juice of 1/2 lemon

4 hard boiled eggs chilled

2 Tablespoons celery

1 Tablespoon chopped parsley

1/2 teaspoon salt

1/4 teaspoon freshly ground pepper

1 head buttercrunch lettuce or 4-5 endive bulbs

1-2 slices cooked bacon

Directions:

In a medium bowl, mash avocado and lemon juice together with a fork until it is creamy and smooth. It's okay if there are still a few lumps.

With a box grater over the bowl, grate in the four hard boiled eggs. Add the chopped celery, parsley, and seasonings to the bowl .

Combine gently with a fork until everything is incorporated. Taste the egg salad and adjust the seasonings as needed. At this point the mixture can be refrigerated for up to 2 hours,

Break off the lettuce or endive leaves and arrange them on a plate. Spoon the egg salad into the lettuce cups and top with chopped bacon and more parsley. Serve at once.

Nutrition:

Calories per serving: 452

Carbohydrates: 2g

Protein: 43g

Fat: 45g

Sugar: 0.1g

Sodium: 155mg

Fiber: 0.7g

Day 5 - Burger In A Lettuce Bun, Accompanied With Avocado And Served With A Side Salad

Preparation Time: 15 minutes

Cooking Time: 25 minutes

Serves: 4

Ingredients:

Sauce:

1/4 cup Greek yogurt

2 tablespoons adobo sauce (from canned chipotles in adobo)

1 tablespoon Dijon mustard

2 dashes Worcestershire sauce

Burgers:

2 pounds ground chuck

1 teaspoon kosher salt

1/2 teaspoon freshly ground black pepper

5 dashes Worcestershire sauce

Toppings:

1 head iceberg, green leaf or butter lettuce

2 avocados, sliced

1 tomato, sliced

1/4 red onion, thinly sliced into rings

12 small sweet pickles, chopped

Directions:

For the sauce: Mix together the yogurt, adobo sauce, mustard and Worcestershire sauce in a small bowl. Set aside.

For the burgers: In a bowl, combine the ground chuck, salt, black pepper and Worcestershire sauce. Form four patties and set aside.

Heat a skillet over medium-high heat. Cook the patties until done in the middle, 4 to 6 minutes per side.

For the toppings: Cut the base of each lettuce leaf on the head and carefully peel it away so that it stays as intact as possible.

Top the patties with avocado slices, tomato slices, red onion rings and chopped pickles, then drizzle with the sauce to taste. Use two or three lettuce leaves per patty and wrap them around the patty as tightly as you can. Slice in half and serve immediately!

Nutrition:

Calories per serving: 548

Carbohydrates: 2g

Protein: 65g

Fat: 39g

Sugar: 0.1g

Sodium: 175mg

Fiber: 0.7g

Day 6 - Poached Salmon And Avocado Rolls Wrapped In Seaweed

Preparation Time: 30 minutes

Cooking Time: 30 minutes

Serves: 2

Ingredients:

1 to 1½ pounds salmon fillets, pin bones removed

Salt

½ cup dry white wine (a good Sauvignon Blanc)

½ cup water

1 shallot, peeled and thinly sliced or a few thin slices of onion

Several sprigs of fresh dill or sprinkle of dried dill

A sprig of fresh parsley

Freshly ground black pepper

A few slices of fresh lemon to serve

4 sheets nori seaweed (available from natural food stores and Japanese markets)

450 grams (1 pound) cucumbers, thinly sliced with a mandolin slicer (I don't peel my cucumbers; see note)

toasted sesame seeds

ground chili powder (optional)

1 ripe avocado, sliced into thin wedges

100 grams (3 1/2 ounces) tofu, or cooked chicken, or fish (raw and super fresh, or cooked), cut into strips

long-stem sprouts or sprouted seeds

soy sauce, for serving

Directions:

1 Sprinkle the salmon fillets with a little salt. Put the wine, water, dill, parsley and shallots or onions in a sauté pan, and bring to a simmer on medium heat.

Place salmon fillets, skin-side down on the pan. Cover. Cook 5 to 10 minutes, depending on the thickness of the fillet, or to desired done-ness. Do not overcook.

Serve sprinkled with freshly ground black pepper and a slice or two of lemon.

Now make the avocado rolls. Have all the ingredients ready and portioned out into four equal servings before you begin, and have a small bowl or glass of water close at hand.

Place a sheet of nori on a clean and dry cutting board, shiny side facing down and longest edge facing you.

Starting from the left edge, arrange the cucumber slices in overlapping rows on the nori, leaving a 3-cm (1-inch) margin of uncovered nori at right.

Sprinkle with sesame and ground chili powder, if using.

If using tahini sauce or cashew cheese, drizzle or smear over the cucumber now.

If using sliced radishes or salad leaves, arrange in a single layer on top of the cucumber now.

Arrange the bulkier fillings -- avocado, tofu, sprouts, herbs, mango, jicama -- in an even, vertical pattern, about 5 cm (2 inches) from the left edge.

Rotate the cutting board by a quarter of a turn counter-clockwise so the uncovered strip of nori is furthest from you. Using both hands, start rolling the sheet of nori from the edge closest to you, folding it up and over the fillings, then rolling it snugly away from you (see note).

Just as you're about to reach the uncovered strip of nori at the end, dip your fingertips in the bowl of water and dab the nori lightly so it will stick.

Set aside, seam side down, and repeat with the remaining ingredients to make three more rolls.

Slice into halves or thick slices using a sharp chef knife. Served together with the poached salmon with soy sauce for dipping.

Nutrition:

Calories per serving: 584

Carbohydrates: 3g

Protein: 52g

Fat: 45g

Sugar: 0.1g

Sodium: 175mg

Fiber: 3g

Day 7 - Tuna Salad Made With Mayo, Served In Avocado Halves

Preparation Time: 15 minutes

Cooking Time: 0 minutes

Serves: 2

Ingredients:

1 can (5.5 ounces) water-packed tuna, drained

2 tablespoon of mayonnaise

2 tablespoon of fresh lemon juice

1 chopped celery stalk

Salt and pepper

2 avocados halve and pitted

Directions:

Combine drained tuna in a small bowl with mayonnaise, lemon juice, and celery. Season with salt and pepper.

Fill each avocado with tuna mixture, evenly divided. Garnish with celery leaves if desired. Serve and Enjoy!

Nutrition:

Calories per serving: 652

Carbohydrates: 1g

Protein: 48g

Fat: 35g

Sugar: 0.1g

Sodium: 145mg

Fiber: 1.5g

Chapter 36: Dinner Recipes from the 7-Day Meal Plan

Day 1 - Garlic And Herb Shrimp In Butter Sauce With Zucchini Noodles

Preparation Time: 15 minutes

Cooking Time: 30 minutes

Serves: 6

Ingredients:

4 tablespoons unsalted butter, divided

4 cloves garlic, minced and divided

1 pound (3 medium-sized) zucchini, spiralized*

Kosher salt and freshly ground black pepper, to taste

1 shallot, minced

1 pound medium shrimp, peeled and deveined

2 teaspoons lemon zest

2 tablespoons chopped fresh parsley leaves

Directions:

Melt 1 tablespoon butter in a large skillet over medium heat. Add 2 cloves garlic and cook, stirring frequently, until fragrant, about 1 minute.

Stir in zucchini noodles until just tender, about 2-3 minutes; season with salt and pepper, to taste. Set aside and keep warm.

Melt the remaining 3 tablespoons butter in the skillet. Add remaining 2 cloves garlic and shallot, and cook, stirring frequently, until fragrant, about 2 minutes.

Add shrimp; season with salt and pepper, to taste. Cook, stirring occasionally, until pink and cooked through, about 3-4 minutes. Stir in lemon zest and parsley.

Serve immediately with zucchini noodles.

Nutrition:

Calories per serving: 352

Carbohydrates: 2g

Protein: 42.5g

Fat: 42g

Sugar: 0.1g

Sodium: 152mg

Fiber: 0.7g

Day 2 - Beef Stew With Mushrooms And Onions

Preparation Time: 15 minutes

Cooking Time: 30 minutes

Serves: 6

Ingredients:

2 lbs. beef sirloin or chuck cut into cubes

1 1/2 teaspoons sea salt

1/4 teaspoon ground black pepper

1/4 cup butter

2 lbs. chopped white mushrooms

1 medium yellow onion chopped

5 cloves garlic crushed

1/4 cup tomato paste

1 can 10 oz. cream of mushroom

4 cups beef broth

2 teaspoons dried parsley flakes

1/2 teaspoon dried oregano

Directions:

Rub salt and ground black pepper on the beef. Let it stay for 10 minutes.

Melt 1 tablespoon butter in a Dutch oven or cooking pot. Put the beef in and cook for 3 to 5 minutes or until the color turns light brown.

Remove the beef. Set Aside. Melt the remaining butter in the same cooking pot.

Once the butter melts, sauté the mushrooms, onions, and garlic. Continue to cook until the mushrooms become soft.

Add the beef. Cook for 2 minutes.

Add the tomato paste, parsley, oregano, and beef broth. Stir and let boil. Cover and simmer 60 min.

Add the cream of mushroom. Stir and cook for 2 to 3 minutes.

Turn the heat off. Transfer to a serving plate. Share and enjoy!

Nutrition:

Calories per serving: 452

Carbohydrates: 2g

Protein: 49g

Fat: 44g

Sugar: 2g

Sodium: 174mg

Fiber: 3g

Day 3 - Grilled Shrimp Topped With Lemon And Served With Broccoli

Preparation Time: 15 minutes

Cooking Time: 30 minutes

Serves: 6

Ingredients:

2 large heads broccoli, trimmed into bite-sized florets

4 tablespoons olive oil, divided

1 teaspoon kosher salt, plus more to taste if desired

1 teaspoon freshly ground black pepper, plus more to taste if desired

1 pound raw shrimp, cleaned, deveined, shells removed (I used U12 shrimp, i.e. 12 per 1 pound)

1/4 cup unsalted butter, melted

1/4 cup freshly squeezed lemon juice

Directions:

Preheat oven to high broiler setting and place the top oven rack about 4 inches below the broiler. Line a half-sheet pan with aluminum foil for easier cleanup, add the broccoli, evenly drizzle with 2 tablespoons olive oil, 1 teaspoon salt, 1 teaspoon pepper, toss with your hands to combine, place sheet pan under the broiler, and broil for about 5 minutes, or until florets are turning lightly browned and dried out looking on the tips of the florets.

Remove pan from the oven, flip and toss the broccoli, add the shrimp, evenly drizzle the shrimp with the remaining 2 teaspoons olive oil, and return pan to the broiler for about 2 to 3 minutes, or until shrimp are cooked through. There is no need to flip them. Remove pan from the oven and set aside.

Melt the butter in a small microwave-safe bowl, add the lemon juice, stir to combine, and evenly drizzle over the shrimp and broccoli, as desired. Taste and check for seasoning balance and add more salt and/or pepper, as desired, and serve immediately. Recipe will keep airtight in the fridge for up to 3 days.

Nutrition:

Calories per serving: 425

Carbohydrates: 6g

Protein: 47g

Fat: 32g

Sugar: 0.1g

Sodium: 162mg

Fiber: 0.7g

Day 4 - Cajun Chicken Breast With Cauliflower Rice And Brussels Sprouts

Preparation Time: 15 minutes

Cooking Time: 40 minutes

Serves: 3

Ingredients:

¼ lb. Chicken Breast

1 tablespoon avocado oil or olive oil

1 small onion, diced

3 cloves garlic, minced

8 cups riced cauliflower

1 cup chicken stock

1 tablespoon plus 2 teaspoons Creole seasoning, more to taste

1 small red bell pepper, diced

1 small green bell pepper, diced

1 small yellow bell pepper, diced

chopped fresh flat-leaf parsley, for garnish

5 ounces Brussel Sprouts

Directions:

Heat the oil in a large skillet over medium heat.

Season strips of chicken breasts with salt and pepper.

Pan fry for 3mins each side or until cooked. Then set aside.

On the same pan, add the onion and garlic and sauté until the onions are translucent and the garlic is fragrant.

Add the cauliflower, and sauté until the cauliflower is tender, about 15 minutes.

Add the stock and the seasoning and cook, stirring often, for an additional 10 to 15 minutes, or until all of the stock is evaporated and the rice is tender but not mushy.

Add the bell peppers and cook an additional 10 minutes.

Blanch Brussel sprouts by boiling water for 5 minutes, followed by an ice bath.

Sauté with garlic and onion. Add fresh lemon juice, Balsamic vinegar and toss so Brussels sprouts are evenly coated or sprinkle with Parmesan cheese.

Add chopped Brussels sprouts to the dish.

Garnish with parsley before serving.

Nutrition:

Calories per serving: 475

Carbohydrates: 2g

Protein: 45g

Fat: 35g

Sugar: 0.1g

Sodium: 172mg

Fiber: 4g

Day 5 - Baked Tofu With Cauliflower Rice, Broccoli, Bell Peppers, And A Thai Peanut Butter Sauce

Preparation Time: 15 minutes

Cooking Time: 45 minutes

Serves: 4

Ingredients:

12 ounces extra-firm tofu

1 tbsp toasted sesame oil

1 small head cauliflower

2 cloves garlic

1 1/2 tbsp toasted sesame oil

1/4 cup low sodium soy sauce

1/4 cup light brown sugar

1/2 tsp chili garlic sauce

2 1/2 tbsp peanut butter or almond butter

Veggies: baby bok choy, green onion, red pepper, broccoli

Toppings: fresh lime juice, cilantro, sriracha

Directions:

Begin by draining tofu 1.5 hours before you want your meal ready. If your block of tofu is larger than 12 ounces, trim it down. You don't need a full pound for this recipe.

Roll tofu in an absorbent towel several times and then place something heavy on top to press. I use a pot on top of a cutting board and sometimes add something to the pot to add more weight. Do this for 15 minutes.

Near the end of draining, preheat oven to 400 degrees F (204 C) and cube tofu. Place on a parchment-lined baking sheet and arrange in a single layer. Bake for 25 minutes to dry/firm the tofu. Once baked, remove from oven and let cool.

Prepare sauce by whisking together ingredients until combined. Taste and adjust flavor as needed. I often add a little more sweetener and peanut butter.

Add cooled tofu to the sauce and stir to coat. Let marinate for at least 15 minutes to saturate the tofu and infuse the flavor.

In the meantime, shred your cauliflower into rice by using a large grater or food processor. You don't want it too fine, just somewhat close to the texture of rice. Set aside. Mince garlic if you haven't already done so, and prepare any veggies you want to add to the dish.

Heat a large skillet over medium to medium-high heat and if adding any veggies to your dish, cook them now in a bit of sesame oil and a dash of soy sauce. Remove from pan and set aside and cover to keep warm.

Use a slotted spoon to spoon tofu into the preheated pan. Add a few spoonful's of the sauce to coat. Cook, stirring frequently for a few minutes until browned. It will stick to the pan a bit, so don't worry. Remove from pan and set aside and cover to keep warm.

Rinse your pan under very hot water and scrape away any residue. Place back on oven.

Add a drizzle of sesame oil to the pan, then add garlic and cauliflower rice and stir. Put cover on to steam the "rice." Cook for about 5-8 minutes until slightly browned and tender, stirring occasionally. Then add a few spoonful's of sauce to season and stir.

Place cauliflower rice and top with veggies and tofu. Serve with any leftover sauce. Leftovers reheat well and will keep covered in the fridge for up to a couple days.

Nutrition:

Calories per serving: 416

Carbohydrates: 6g

Protein: 47g

Fat: 32g

Sugar: 0.1g

Sodium: 162mg

Fiber: 9g

Day 6 - Grilled Beef Kebabs With Peppers And Broccoli

Preparation Time: 20 minutes

Cooking Time: 35 minutes

Serves: 4

Ingredients:

1/3 c. low-sodium soy sauce

1/4 c. brown sugar

Juice of 2 limes (or 1 if large), plus more for serving

1 tbsp. ground ginger

1 lb. sirloin steak, cut into cubes

2 c. broccoli florets

2 tbsp. extra-virgin olive oil

Freshly ground black pepper

Green onions, for garnish

Directions:

Heat grill to medium-high. In a small bowl, whisk together soy sauce, brown sugar, lime juice and ginger.

Add steak and toss until coated. Let marinate in the fridge, at least 15 minutes and up 2 hours.

In another bowl, toss broccoli florets with olive oil.

Skewer steak and broccoli and season all over with pepper.

Grill, turning occasionally, until steak is medium, 8 minutes.

Squeeze with lime, garnish with green onions, and serve.

Nutrition:

Calories per serving: 321

Carbohydrates: 3g

Protein: 53g

Fat: 25g

Sugar: 0.1g

Sodium: 132mg

Fiber: 3g

Day 7 - Trout Broiled With Butter And Sautéed Bok Choy

Preparation Time: 15 minutes

Cooking Time: 30 minutes

Serves: 6

Ingredients:

1/2 tablespoon honey

1 tablespoon tamari

1 large garlic clove, minced

3/4 teaspoon chili powder

1 filet (6 ounce) trout fish (skin on)

Sea salt, to taste

Fresh ground black pepper to taste

2 heads baby bok choy, rinsed and halved

1/2 teaspoon sesame oil

1/4 teaspoon hot pepper flakes

Directions:

Preheat oven to 425 degrees Fahrenheit and line a baking sheet with parchment paper.

In a bowl, whisk together the honey, half the tamari, minced garlic and chili powder; stir well to mix.

Lay the rainbow trout skin side down onto parchment paper and season with salt and pepper. Use a brush to spread the honey garlic mixture onto the fish.

Add the bok choy to a large mixing bowl and drizzle with the remaining tamari and sesame oil. Toss well.

Transfer bok choy to baking sheet and organize it around the rainbow trout.

Place in the oven and bake for 12 to 15 minutes or until the fish flakes easily when poked with a fork.

Remove from oven and enjoy.

Nutrition:

Calories per serving: 352

Carbohydrates: 2g

Protein: 42.5g

Fat: 42g

Sugar: 0.1g

Sodium: 150mg

Fiber: 0.7g

Chapter 37: Keto Breakfast Recipes

1. Biscuits and Gravy

Preparation Time: 15 minutes

Cooking Time: 1 hour

Serves: 6

Ingredients:

¼ tsp. sea salt

¼ tsp. xanthan gum*

½ tsp. garlic powder

1 tbsp. baking powder

2 lg. eggs

3 c. almond flour, finely ground

6 tbsp. butter softened

¼ tsp. xanthan gum*

½ c. chicken broth

½ c. heavy whipping cream

½ tsp. black pepper, ground

½ tsp. sea salt

1 lb. ground breakfast sausage

2 oz. cream cheese

2 tbsp. butter

Directions:

Preheat the oven to 400° Fahrenheit and line a baking sheet with parchment paper.

In a large mixing bowl, combine all the dry ingredients Directions: biscuits and whisk together.

Add softened butter and the eggs to the dry ingredients and whisk until completely mixed.

Gently form the dough into 10 biscuit shapes with your hands and place them one to two inches apart on the baking sheet.

Bake for 12 to 14 minutes, just until the tops begin to take on a golden brown color.

Let cool completely.

Warm a skillet over medium heat and brown the breakfast sausage completely, breaking it up into smaller pieces as you do so.

Add the butter and cream cheese to the skillet and stir until completely combined. This could take a few minutes to reach an even texture.

Add the cream and broth to the pan and continue to mix, then add the xanthan gum, salt, and pepper and mix once more.

Heat the mixture until it reaches a low boil, then kill the heat. Stir with the heat off until it starts to thicken into a gravy.

Serve warm over the biscuits!

*This is used to thicken the stew but can be substituted for arrowroot, cornstarch, or flour. Chef's choice!

Calories per serving: 521

Carbohydrates: 5g

Protein: 42g

Fat: 46g

Sugar: 0.1g

Sodium: 165mg

Fiber: 0.7g

2. Banana Nut Muffins

Preparation Time: 15 minutes

Cooking Time: 20 minutes

Serves: 7

Ingredients:

¼ c. almond flour

¼ c. almond milk, unsweetened

¼ c. sour cream

½ c. erythritol, or equal measure of preferred sweetener

½ tsp. cinnamon, ground

1 tsp. vanilla extract

2 ½ tsp. banana extract

2 lg. eggs

2 tbsp. flaxseed, ground

2 tsp. baking powder

5 tbsp. butter, melted

Directions:

¾ c. walnuts, chopped

1 tbsp. almond flour

1 tbsp. butter, chilled and cubed

1 tbsp. erythritol, powdered, or equal measure of preferred powdered sweetener.

Preheat the oven to 350° Fahrenheit and fill a muffin tin with muffin liners.

In a large mixing bowl, combine sweetener, almond flour, flaxseed, cinnamon, and baking powder. Whisk until completely combined.

Stir in the melted butter, extracts, almond milk, and sour cream. Add the eggs to the mixture and mix until completely combined.

Fill each tin about ¾ of the way and set aside.

Combine nuts, almond flour, and butter in the food processor and pulse until the nuts are chopped into small pieces. If the mixture seems a little too dry, you may add more butter to moisten it.

Sprinkle the mixture evenly over the tops of all the muffin tins.

Sprinkle the sweetener over each muffin.

Bake for 20 minutes, or until they've taken on a golden brown color and an inserted toothpick comes out clean.

Let cool for 30 minutes or more to cool and firm.

Enjoy!

Calories per serving: 545

Carbohydrates: 2g

Protein: 47g

Fat: 34g

Sugar: 0.1g

Sodium: 175mg

Fiber: 0.7g

3. Egg Cups with Mushrooms

Preparation Time: 15 minutes

Cooking Time: 20 minutes

Serves: 5

Ingredients:

¼ c. almond milk, unsweetened

1/3 c. feta cheese crumbles

½ tbsp. extra virgin olive oil

10 slices bacon

2 cloves garlic, minced

3 c. baby leaf spinach

6 lg. eggs

8 oz. mushrooms, sliced

Sea salt & pepper, to taste

Directions:

Preheat the oven to 400° Fahrenheit and line 10 wells of a muffin tin with a slice of bacon, pressing it gently to the sides. You'll notice some overlapping, which is perfectly fine.

Bake for 15 minutes to allow it to partially cook.

Heat a large skillet over medium heat and warm the olive oil in it. Once warm, add the mushrooms and garlic, sautéing them for about five minutes.

Once the mushrooms gain a bit of color, add the spinach into the pan and stir to wilt it, then set aside off the burner.

In a mixing bowl, combine the eggs, almond milk, and salt & pepper. Whisk until completely combined and pull the muffin tin out of the oven.

You may find that you have excess grease to dispose of from the muffin tin. You can soak up the grease with a paper towel, or you can pull the bacon out of the wells, turn it upside down to drain, then set the bacon back into the cups. If you decide to completely wipe out the grease from the pan, spritz it with a little non-stick spray before putting the bacon back into the tin.

Evenly put the veggies into each tin, then pour the egg mixture over top of it to fill each one most of the way.

Bake for 15 to 20 minutes, or until the tops are golden.

Cool for about five minutes before freeing the cups from the tin by running a butter knife along the edges gently.

Calories per serving: 512

Carbohydrates: 2g

Protein: 45g

Fat: 41g

Sugar: 0.1g

Sodium: 178mg

Fiber: 0.7g

4. Green Smoothie

Preparation Time: 15 minutes

Cooking Time: 0 minutes

Serves: 6

Ingredients:

1 ½ c. ice

1 med. banana

2 handfuls baby leaf spinach

½ avocado

1 ½ c. almond milk, unsweetened

2 scoops protein powder

Directions:

Combine all ingredients into a blender.

Blend until very smooth.

Serve chilled and enjoy!

Calories per serving: 452

Carbohydrates: 2g

Protein: 43g

Fat: 45g

Sugar: 0.1g

Sodium: 155mg

Fiber: 0.7g

5. Coconut Pancakes

Preparation Time: 15 minutes

Cooking Time: 20 minutes

Serves: 5

Calories: 96 | Fat: 7g | Carbohydrates: 3g | Protein: 3g

Ingredients:

1/8 tsp. sea salt

¼ c. coconut flour

1 tsp. baking powder

1 tsp. vanilla extract

2 tbsp. extra virgin olive oil

2 tbsp. maple syrup

3 lg. eggs

Directions:

In a large mixing bowl, combine coconut flour, olive oil, eggs, maple syrup, vanilla extract, salt, and baking powder. Stir thoroughly using a whisk and break up any clumps as you go.

Heat a skillet over medium heat and grease it using more olive oil or your preferred fat source.

Spoon the batter into the skillet about ¼ cup at a time and allow to cook for about four to five minutes until bubbles form in the center of the pancake, then flip and cook for another four to five minutes.

Repeat until you're out of batter and serve warm!

Calories per serving: 352

Carbohydrates: 2g

Protein: 42.5g

Fat: 42g

Sugar: 0.1g

Sodium: 152mg

Fiber: 0.7g

6. Spinach Artichoke Breakfast Bake

Preparation Time: 15 minutes

Cooking Time: 20 minutes

Serves: 7

Ingredients:

¼ c. milk, fat-free

¼ tsp. ground pepper

1/3 c. red pepper, diced

½ c. feta cheese crumbles

½ c. scallions, finely sliced

¾ c. canned artichokes, chopped, drained, & patted dry

1 ¼ tsp. kosher salt

1 clove garlic, minced

1 tbsp. dill, chopped

10 oz. spinach, frozen, chopped & drained

2 tbsp. parmesan cheese, grated

4 lg. egg whites

8 lg. eggs

Directions:

Preheat the oven to 375° Fahrenheit and grease a large baking dish with nonstick spray or preferred fat source.

In a small bowl, combine the spinach, artichoke, scallions, garlic, red pepper, and fill. Combine completely and then pour into the baking dish, spreading into an even layer.

In a mixing bowl, combine eggs, egg whites, salt, pepper, parmesan, and milk. Whisk until completely combined, then add feta and mix once more.

Pour the egg mixture evenly over the vegetables in the baking dish.

Bake for about 35 minutes, until a butter knife inserted in the center comes out clean.

Allow to cool for about 10 minutes before cutting into eight equal pieces.

Serve warm!

Calories per serving: 574

Carbohydrates: 2g

Protein: 47g

Fat: 54g

Sugar: 0.1g

Sodium: 254mg

Fiber: 0.7g

7. Granola Bars

Preparation Time: 15 minutes

Cooking Time: 20 minutes

Serves: 6

Ingredients:

2 c. almonds, chopped

½ c. pumpkin seeds, raw

1/3 c. coconut flakes, unsweetened

2 tbsp. hemp seeds

¼ c. clear Sukrin Fiber Syrup

¼ c. almond butter

¼ c. erythritol, powdered, or equal measure of preferred sweetener

2 tsp. vanilla extract

1/2 tsp. sea salt

Directions:

Line a small, square baking dish with parchment paper.

In a mixing bowl, combine almonds, pumpkin seeds, coconut flakes, and hemp seeds. Stir until evenly mixed.

Over medium heat, combine the syrup, almond butter, sweetener, and salt and stir until it's smooth and easy to pull the spoon through.

Remove the pan from the heat and stir the vanilla extract into the mixture.

Pour the syrup over the seeds and stir completely.

Pour the mixture into the baking dish and press evenly into one layer and press until the top is even.

Let cool completely and slice into 12 bars.

Calories per serving: 254

Carbohydrates: 2g

Protein: 42.5g

Fat: 47g

Sugar: 0.1g

Sodium: 145mg

Fiber: 0.7g

8. Banana Bread

Preparation Time: 15 minutes

Cooking Time: 20 minutes

Serves: 7

Ingredients:

¼ c. almond milk, unsweetened

¼ c. coconut flour

¼ tsp. sea salt

½ c. erythritol, or equal measure of preferred sweetener

½ c. walnuts, chopped

½ tsp. xanthan gum*

2 c. almond flour

2 tsp. baking powder

2 tsp. banana extract

2 tsp. cinnamon, ground

4 lg. eggs

6 tbsp. butter softened

Directions:

Preheat the oven to 350° Fahrenheit and line a loaf pan with parchment paper.

In a large mixing bowl, combine the flours, baking powder, sea salt, and cinnamon and mix thoroughly.

In another bowl, cream the butter and the sweetener with a hand mixer. Beat the eggs into the mixture and then do the same with both the vanilla and the banana extracts.

Pour the dry ingredients into the wet and mix on low with your hand or stand mixer until a batter begins to form.

Mix the chopped walnuts into the mixture.

Pour the batter into the loaf pan and sprinkle more walnuts onto the top.

Bake for about an hour, or until the top is slightly golden and an inserted toothpick comes out clean.

Allow to cool completely before slicing into 12 pieces.

Serve!

*This is used to thicken the stew but can be substituted for arrowroot, cornstarch, or flour. Chef's choice!

Calories per serving: 245

Carbohydrates: 4g

Protein: 47g

Fat: 22g

Sugar: 2g

Sodium: 125mg

Fiber: 0.7g

Chapter 38: Keto Lunch Recipes

9. Carpaccio

Preparation time: 10 minutes

Cooking time: 10 minutes

Servings: 2

Ingredients:

100 grams of smoked prime rib

30 grams of arugula

20 grams of Parmesan cheese

10 grams of pine nuts

7 grams of butter

3 tablespoons of olive oil with orange

1 tablespoon of lemon juice

Pepper and salt

Directions:

Arrange the meat slices on a plate.

Place meat products on a plate

Wash the arugula and pat dry or use a salad spinner.

Place the arugula on top of the meat.

Place arugula on the meat

Scrape some curls from the Parmesan cheese and spread them over the arugula.

Spread Parmesan cheese over the arugula

Put the butter in a small frying pan. Add the pine nuts as soon as the butter has melted. Let the pine nuts bake for a few minutes over a medium heat and then sprinkle them over the carpaccio.

Sprinkle pine nuts over the carpaccio

Make vinaigrette by mixing the lemon juice into the olive oil. Season with pepper and salt and drizzle over the carpaccio.

Nutrition:

Calories: 350 kcal

Gross carbohydrates: 3 g

Protein: 31 g | Fat: 24 g

Fiber: 1 g

Net carbohydrates: 2 g

Macro fat: 42 %

Macro proteins: 54 %

Macro carbohydrates: 4 %

10. Keto Spring Frittata

Preparation time: 5 minutes

Cooking time: 10 minutes

Servings: 2

Ingredients:

1 zucchini

0.5 bunch of mint

6 eggs

pinch of cayenne pepper

1 sprig of thyme or 1 teaspoon of dried thyme

80 grams of Pecorino cheese

0.5 red chili pepper

100 grams of feta cheese

3 tablespoons of extra virgin olive oil

0.25 teaspoon truffle oil optional

Salt to taste

Salad

50 grams of watercress

0.5 stalk of celery

75 grams of fresh (raw) peas still in the pod

1 tablespoon of lemon juice

2 tablespoons of extra virgin olive oil

Herb cheese or boursin

200 grams of herb cheese or boursin

Directions:

If you have an oven with a grill, turn the grill on at the highest setting.

Grate the zucchini by hand or in the food processor and put in a bowl. Sprinkle some salt over the grated zucchini.

Put the zucchini in a strainer and press the zucchini firmly so that some of the moisture goes out.

Wash the mint and pat dry. Remove the leaves from the twigs and cut them into pieces. Add to the zucchini and mix together.

Heat the olive oil in a small (frying) pan over a medium-high heat. Add the zucchini as soon as the oil is hot and spread over the pan. Lower the heat to moderate.

Spread the zucchini over the pan

Beat the eggs in the bowl and add the truffle oil, cayenne pepper and thyme leaves. Grate the pecorino and add half of the pecorino to the bowl.

Beat eggs with thyme and cayenne pepper and truffle oil

Pour the beaten eggs over the zucchini in the frying pan. Mix in the zucchini. Reduce the heat and simmer for 5 minutes while making the salad.

Put the frittata in a baking dish or on a large plate and sprinkle the rest of the pecorino over it. Place as high as possible in the oven, just below the grill and brown for 5 minutes. If you don't have a grill, let the frittata cook on the stove for 5 minutes with a lid on the pan, if you want the cheese to melt, you can gently turn the frittata by putting a lid or plate on the pan and then turning it over.

Spring frittata under the grill

Wash the chili pepper and remove the seeds. Cut into small rings and sprinkle over the frittata as soon as it comes out of the oven. Also crumble the feta over the frittata.

Spring frittata from Jamie Oliver

Salad

Bring a saucepan of water to the boil and add a pinch of salt.

Wash the watercress and pat dry. Put in a salad bowl. Wash the celery and cut into 5 cm pieces and cut them into thin sticks (also use the celery leaves).

Remove the peas from the cap and blanch them for 1-2 minutes in the boiling water in the saucepan (the same applies to frozen peas or snow peas). Then let them drain in a colander. If you have fresh peas from the pod, this is not necessary.

While the peas are cooling down, make vinaigrette by mixing lemon juice with the extra virgin olive oil.

Add the peas to the salad and pour the vinaigrette over it. Mix everything together very well.

Nutrition:

Calories: 955 kcal

Gross carbohydrates: 16 g

Protein: 46 g

Fats: 78 g

Fiber: 2 g

Net carbohydrates: 14 g

Macro fats: 57 %

Macro proteins: 33 %

Macro carbohydrates: 10 %

11. Super-Fast Keto Sandwiches

Preparation time: 5 minutes

Cooking time: 5 minutes

Servings: 1 sandwich

Ingredients:

1 teaspoon of hemp flour

1 teaspoon of almond flour

1 teaspoon of psyllium

1 teaspoon of baking powder

1 egg at room temperature

1 teaspoon of extra virgin olive oil or melted butter

Directions:

Put the dry ingredients in a cup and mix well. In particular, ensure that the baking powder is no longer visible. It helps if you put the baking powder through a (tea) strainer.

Now add the egg and the butter. The egg must be at room temperature. If it is not, then place it for about 10 minutes in a bowl with hot tap water.

Stir well and let it stand for a while. You will see that there are some bubbles in the batter.

Now put the cup in the microwave for 1 minute on the highest setting. When you take the cup out, you want the top of the batter to be dry. If it is still wet, then put it in the microwave for a little longer. (If you put several cups in the microwave at the same time, you may have to extend the time slightly depending on your type of microwave).

Once the top is dry, remove the cup from the microwave and turn it on a cutting board. Decide now if you want thick rolls or something thinner. So cut into 2 or 3 or 4 slices. Keep in mind that these slices must fit in your toaster.

Now toast the bread slices in your toaster until they are firm but not hard.

Your bread is now ready. You can use it immediately or use it for your breakfast or lunch the another day. Spread the butter on it well so that you will get enough fats.

Nutrition:

Calories: 112 kcal

Gross carbohydrates: 2 g

Protein: 9 g

Fats: 6 g

Fiber: 5 g

Net carbohydrates: -3 g

Macro fat: 50 %

Macro proteins: 75 %

Macro carbohydrates: -25 %

12. Keto Croque Monsieur

Preparation time: 5 minutes

Cooking time: 7 minutes

Servings: 2

Ingredients:

2 eggs

25 grams of grated cheese

25 grams of ham 1 large slice

40 ml of cream

40 ml of mascarpone

30 grams of butter

Pepper and salt

Basil leaves, optional, to garnish

Directions:

Carefully crack eggs in a neat bowl, add some salt and pepper.

Add the cream, mascarpone and grated cheese and stir together.

Melt the butter over a medium heat. The butter must not turn brown. Once the butter has melted, set the heat to low.

Add half of the omelette mixture to the frying pan and then immediately place the slice of ham on it. Now pour the rest of the omelette mixture over the ham and then immediately put a lid on it.

Allow it to fry for 2-3 minutes over a low heat until the top is slightly firmer.

Slide the omelette onto the lid to turn the omelette. Then put the omelette back in the frying pan to fry for another 1-2 minutes on the other side (still on low heat), then put the lid back on the pan.

Don't let the omelette cook for too long! It does not matter if it is still liquid. Garnish with a few basil leaves if necessary.

Nutrition:

Calories: 479 kcal

Gross carbohydrates: 4 g

Protein: 16 g

Fats: 45 g

Net carbohydrates: 4 g

Macro fats: 69 %

Macro proteins: 25 %

Macro carbohydrates: 6 %

13. Keto Wraps With Cream Cheese And Salmon

Preparation time: 5 minutes

Cooking time: 10 minutes

Servings: 2

Ingredients:

80 grams of cream cheese

1 tablespoon of dill or other fresh herbs

30 grams of smoked salmon

1 egg

15 grams of butter

Pinch of cayenne pepper

Pepper and salt

Directions:

Beat the egg well in a bowl. With 1 egg, you can make two thin wraps in a small frying pan.

Melt the butter over a medium heat in a small frying pan. Once the butter has melted, add half of the beaten egg to the pan. Move the pan back and forth so that the entire bottom is covered with a very thin layer of egg. Turn down the heat!

Carefully loosen the egg on the edges with a silicone spatula and turn the wafer-thin omelette as soon as the egg is no longer dripping (about 45 seconds to 1 minute). You can do this by sliding it onto a lid or plate and then sliding it back into the pan. Let the other side be cooked for about 30 seconds and then remove from the pan. The omelette must be nice and light yellow. Repeat for the rest of the beaten egg.

Once the omelettes are ready, let them cool on a cutting board or plate and make the filling.

Cut or cut the dill into small pieces and put in a bowl.

Add the cream cheese and the salmon, cut into small pieces. Mix together. Add a tiny bit of cayenne pepper and mix well. Taste immediately and then season with salt and pepper.

Spread a layer on the wrap and roll it up. Cut the wrap in half and keep in the fridge until you are ready to eat it.

Nutrition:

Calories: 237

Carbohydrates: 14.7g

Protein: 15g

Fat: 5g

14. Slow Cooker Chilli

Preparation time: 15 minutes

Cooking time: 6 hours and 15 minutes

Servings: 6 servings

Ingredients:

2 ½ lbs ground beef

1 red onion, diced

5 cloves garlic, minced

1 ½ c celery, diced

1 6-ounce can tomato paste

1 14.5 oz can diced tomatoes with green chilies

1 14.5 oz can stewed tomatoes

4 T chili powder

2 T ground cumin

2 t salt

1 t garlic powder

1 t onion powder

3 t cayenne pepper

1 t red pepper flakes

Directions:

Cook ground beef in a large skillet.

Add onion, garlic, and celery and cook until ground beef browned

Drain the fat from the beef

Place beef and vegetable mixture into the slow cooker set on a low setting.

Add tomatoes and seasonings then stir to mix.

Place the lid on the slow cooker and cook on low for 6 hours.

Serve with cheese on top if desired. Adjust the red pepper to taste.

Nutrition:

Calories: 137

Carbohydrates: 4.7g

Protein: 16g

Fat: 5g

Chapter 39: Keto Dinner Recipes

15. Slow Roasting Pork Shoulder

Preparation Time: 15 minutes

Cooking Time: 7 hours

Serves: 8

Ingredients:

3 lb. pork shoulder

8 garlic cloves, minced

½ C. fresh lemon juice

2 tbsp. olive oil

1 tbsp. low-sodium soy sauce

1/3 C. homemade chicken broth

Directions:

In a nonreactive baking dish, arrange the pork shoulder, fat side up.

With the tip of knife, score the fat in a crosshatch pattern.

In a bowl, add the garlic, lemon juice, soy sauce and oil and mix well.

Place the marinade over pork and coat well.

Refrigerate for about 4-6 hours, flipping occasionally.

Preheat the oven to 315o F. Lightly, grease a large roasting pan.

With paper towels, wipe marinade off the pork shoulder.

Arrange the pork shoulder into prepared roasting pan, fat side up.

Roast for about 3 hours.

Remove from the oven and pour the broth over the pork shoulder.

Roast for about 3-4 hours, basting with pan juices, after every 1 hour.

Remove from oven and place the pork shoulder onto a cutting board for about 30 minutes.

With a sharp knife, cut the pork shoulder into desired size slices and serve.

Nutrition:

Calories per serving: 537

Carbohydrates: 1.5g

Protein: 40.2g

Fat: 40.1g

Sugar: 0.5g

Sodium: 261mg

Fiber: 0.1g

16. Garlicky Pork Shoulder

Preparation Time: 15 minutes

Cooking Time: 6 hours

Serves: 10

Ingredients:

1 head garlic, peeled and crushed

¼ C. fresh rosemary, minced

2 tbsp. fresh lemon juice

2 tbsp. balsamic vinegar

1 (4-lb.) pork shoulder

Directions:

In a bowl, add all the ingredients except pork shoulder and mix well.

In a large roasting pan, place the pork shoulder and generously coat with the marinade.

With a large plastic wrap, cover the roasting pan and refrigerate to marinate for at least 1-2 hours.

Remove the roasting pan from refrigerator.

Remove the plastic wrap from roasting pan and keep in room temperature for 1 hour.

Preheat the oven to 2750 F.

Place the roasting pan into oven and roast for about 6 hours.

Remove from the oven and place pork shoulder onto a cutting board for about 30 minutes.

With a sharp knife, cut the pork shoulder into desired size slices and serve.

Nutrition:

Calories per serving: 502

Carbohydrates: 2g

Protein: 42.5g

Fat: 39.1g

Sugar: 0.1g

Sodium: 125mg

Fiber: 0.7g

17. Rosemary Pork Roast

Preparation Time: 15 minutes

Cooking Time: 1 hour

Serves: 6

Ingredients:

1 tbsp. dried rosemary, crushed

3 garlic cloves, minced

Salt and freshly ground black pepper, to taste

2 lb. boneless pork loin roast

¼ C. olive oil

1/3 C. homemade chicken broth

Directions:

Preheat the oven to 3500 F. Lightly, grease a roasting pan.

In a small bowl, add rosemary, garlic, salt and black pepper and with the back of spoon, crush the mixture to form a paste.

With a sharp knife, pierce the pork loin at many places.

Press the half of rosemary mixture into the cuts.

Add oil in the bowl with remaining rosemary mixture and stir to combine.

Rub the pork with rosemary mixture generously.

Arrange the pork loin into the prepared roasting pan.

Roast for about 1 hour, flipping and coating with the pan juices occasionally.

Remove the roasting pan from oven. Transfer the pork into a serving platter.

Place the roasting pan over medium heat.

Add the broth and cook for about 3-5 minutes, stirring to lose the brown bits from pan.

Pour sauce over pork and serve.

Nutrition:

Calories per serving: 294

Carbohydrates: 0.9g

Protein: 40g

Fat: 13.9g

Sugar: 0.1g

Sodium: 156mg

Fiber: 0.3g

18. Winter Season Pork Dish

Preparation Time: 15 minutes

Cooking Time: 2 hours

Serves: 8

Serves: 8 , Cooking Time: 2 hours 12 minutes , Preparation Time: 15 minutes

Ingredients:

24 oz. sauerkraut

2 lb. pork roast

Salt and freshly ground black pepper, to taste

¼ C. unsalted butter

½ yellow onion, sliced thinly

14 oz. precooked kielbasa, sliced into ½-inch rounds

Directions:

Preheat the oven to 3250 F.

Drain the sauerkraut, reserving about 1 C. of liquid.

Lightly, season the pork roast with salt and black pepper.

In a heavy-bottomed skillet, melt the butter over high heat and sear the pork for about 5-6 minutes per side.

With a slotted spoon, transfer the pork onto a plate.

In the bottom of a casserole, place half of sauerkraut and onion slices.

Place the seared pork roast and kielbasa pieces on top.

Top with the remaining sauerkraut and onion slices.

Pour the reserved sauerkraut liquid into casserole dish.

Cover the casserole dish tightly and bake for about 2 hours.

Remove from the oven and with tongs, transfer the pork roast onto a cutting board for at least 15 minutes.

With a sharp knife, cut the pork roast into desired size slices.

Divide the pork slices onto serving plates and serve alongside the sauerkraut mixture.

Nutrition:

Calories per serving: 417

Carbohydrates: 6.3g

Protein: 39g

Fat: 25g

Sugar: 2g

Sodium: 1200mg

Fiber: 3g

19. Celebrating Pork Tenderloin

Preparation Time: 15 minutes

Cooking Time: 40 minutes

Serves: 6

Serves: 6 , Cooking Time: 38 minutes , Preparation Time: 15 minutes

Ingredients:

For Pork Tenderloin:

3 medium garlic cloves, minced

3 tsp. dried rosemary, crushed

½ tsp. cayenne pepper

Salt and freshly ground black pepper, to taste

2 lb. pork tenderloin

For Blueberry Sauce:

1 tbsp. olive oil

1 medium yellow onion, chopped

½ tsp. Erythritol

1/3 C. organic apple cider vinegar

1½ C. fresh blueberries

½ tsp. dried thyme, crushed

Salt and freshly ground black pepper, to taste

Directions:

Preheat the oven to 4000 F. Grease a roasting pan.

For pork: in a bowl, mix together all the ingredients except pork.

Rub the pork with garlic mixture evenly.

Place the pork into prepared roasting pan.

Roast for about 25 minutes or until desired doneness.

Meanwhile, for sauce; in a pan, heat the oil over medium-high heat and sauté the onion for about 4-5 minutes.

Stir in the remaining ingredients and cook for about 7-8 minutes or until desired thickness, stirring frequently.

Remove the roasting pan from oven and place the pork tenderloin onto a cutting board for about 10-15 minutes.

With a sharp knife, cut the pork tenderloin into desired size slices and serve with the topping of blueberry sauce.

Nutrition:

Calories per serving: 276

Carbohydrates: 9g

Protein: 40g

Fat: 8g

Sugar: 5g

Sodium: 116mg

Fiber: 2g

20. Mustard Pork Tenderloin

Preparation Time: 15 minutes

Cooking Time: 30 minutes

Serves: 4

Serves: 4 , Cooking Time: 22 minutes , Preparation Time: 15 minutes

Ingredients:

1 tsp. fresh rosemary, minced

1 garlic clove, minced

1 tbsp. fresh lemon juice

1 tbsp. olive oil

1 tsp. Dijon mustard

1 tsp. powdered Swerve

Salt and freshly ground black pepper, to taste

1 lb. pork tenderloin

¼ C. blue cheese, crumbled

Directions:

Preheat oven to 4000 F. Grease a large rimmed baking sheet.

In a large bowl, add all the ingredients except the pork tenderloin and cheese and beat until well combined.

Add the pork tenderloin and coat with the mixture generously.

Arrange the pork tenderloin onto the prepared baking sheet.

Bake for about 20-22 minutes.

Remove from the oven and place the pork tenderloin onto a cutting board for about 5 minutes.

With a sharp knife, cut the pork tenderloin into ¾-inch thick slices and serve with the topping of cheese.

Nutrition:

Calories per serving: 227

Carbohydrates: 2g

Protein: 37g

Fat: 10g

Sugar: 0.5g

Sodium: 236mg

Fiber: 0.1g

21. Succulent Pork Tenderloin

Preparation Time: 20 minutes

Cooking Time: 1 hour

Serves: 4

Ingredients:

1 lb. pork tenderloin

1 tbsp. unsalted butter

2 tsp. garlic, minced

2 oz. fresh spinach

4 oz. cream cheese, softened

1 tsp. liquid smoke

Salt and freshly ground black pepper, to taste

Directions:

Preheat the oven to 350o F. Line casserole dish with a piece of the foil.

Arrange the pork tenderloin between 2 plastic wraps and with a meat tenderizer, pound until flat.

Carefully, cut the edges of tenderloin to shape into a rectangle.

In a large skillet, melt the butter over medium heat and sauté the garlic for about 1 minute.

Add the spinach, cream cheese, liquid smoke, salt and black pepper and cook for about 3-4 minutes.

Remove from the heat and set aside to cool slightly.

Place the spinach mixture onto pork tenderloin about ½-inch from the edges.

Carefully roll tenderloin into a log and secure with toothpicks.

Arrange the tenderloin into the prepared casserole dish, seam-side down.

Bake for about 1¼ hours.

Remove from the oven and let it cool slightly before cutting.

Cut the tenderloin into desired sized slices and serve.

Nutrition:

Calories per serving: 315

Carbohydrates: 3g

Protein: 43g

Fat: 23g

Sugar: 0.5g

Sodium: 261mg

Fiber: 0.1g

22. Simple Ever Rib Roast

Preparation Time: 15 minutes

Cooking Time: 1 hour

Serves: 15

Ingredients:

10 garlic cloves, minced

2 tsp. dried thyme, crushed

2 tbsp. olive oil

Salt and freshly ground black pepper, to taste

1 (10-lb.) grass-fed prime rib roast

Directions:

In a bowl, mix together all the ingredients except rib roast.

In a large roasting pan, place the rib roast, fatty side up.

Coat the rib roast with garlic mixture evenly.

Set aside to marinate at the room temperature for at least 1 hour.

Preheat the oven to 5000 F.

Roast for about 20 minutes.

Now, reduce the temperature of oven to 3250 F.

Roast for 65-75 minutes.

Remove from oven and place the roast onto a cutting board for about 10-15 minutes before slicing.

With a sharp knife cut the rib roast in desired sized slices and serve.

Nutrition:

Calories per serving: 500

Carbohydrates: 1g

Protein: 60g

Fat: 26g

Sugar: 0.5g

Sodium: 200mg

Fiber: 0.1g

23. Family Dinner Tenderloin

Preparation Time: 15 minutes

Cooking Time: 30 minutes

Serves: 6

Ingredients:

4 garlic cloves, minced

½ C. fresh parsley, chopped

1/3 C. fresh oregano, chopped

2 tbsp. fresh thyme, chopped

2 tbsp. fresh rosemary, chopped

2 tsp. fresh lemon zest, grated

6 tbsp. olive oil

2 tbsp. fresh lemon juice

½ tsp. red pepper flakes

Salt and freshly ground black pepper, to taste

1¾ lb. grass-fed beef tenderloin, silver skin removed

Directions:

In a large bowl, add all the ingredients except the beef tenderloin and mix well.

Add the beef tenderloin and coat with the herb mixture generously.

Refrigerate to marinate for about 30-45 minutes.

Preheat the oven to 4250 F.

Remove the beef tenderloin from the bowl and arrange onto a baking sheet.

Bake for about 30 minutes.

Remove from the oven and place the beef tenderloin onto a cutting board for about 15-20 minutes before slicing.

With a sharp knife, cut the beef tenderloin into desired sized slices and serve.

Nutrition:

Calories per serving: 420

Carbohydrates: 5.2g

Protein: 40g

Fat: 27g

Sugar: 0.5g

Sodium: 121mg

Fiber: 3g

Chapter 40: The Summer Smoothies That Make You Healthy And Beautiful.

24. Coconut Green Smoothie

This smoothie has coconut oil and coconut milk as a wonderful pick-me-up when you need a shot of fiber. Enjoy the fresh coconut flavor that is balanced with matcha. It is a refreshing drink for any time.

Preparation Time: 15 minutes

Cooking Time: 30 minutes

Serves: 6

Ingredients:

⅔ c slightly defrosted frozen chopped spinach

½ avocado

1 T coconut oil

½ t matcha powder

1 T monk fruit sweetener

½ c coconut milk (from the dairy section, not canned)

⅔ c water

½ cup of ice

Directions:

Add all ingredients except the ice into a blender. Blend until everything is blended well.

Pulse in the ice until it is evenly distributed.

Pour into a glass.

This smoothie is good for fiber and fat. You can add flaxseed or softened chia seeds to the smoothie for additional fiber and nutrients. Fresh spinach can be used and may be substituted with fresh or frozen kale.

Nutrition:

Calories per serving: 315

Carbohydrates: 3g

Protein: 43g

Fat: 23g

Sugar: 0.5g

Sodium: 261mg

Fiber: 0.1g

25. Strawberry Smoothie

Add a touch of sweetness to your day with this strawberry smoothie. This smoothie is good enough for dessert. If you want to add some fiber and protein, try adding chia seeds that have been softened in water. 2 tablespoons of chia will add 139 calories, 1 gram of carbohydrate, 4 grams of protein, and 9 grams of fat.

Preparation Time: 15 minutes

Cooking Time: 30 minutes

Serves: 6

Ingredients:

¼ c heavy cream

¾ c unsweetened vanilla almond milk

2 t stevia

½ c frozen strawberries (whole or sliced)

½ c ice (preferably crushed)

Directions:

Blend ingredients in a blender until blended well.

Pour into a tall glass.

Serve.

Nutrition:

Calories per serving: 352

Carbohydrates: 2g

Protein: 42.5g

Fat: 42g

Sugar: 0.1g

Sodium: 152mg

Fiber: 0.7g

26. Keto Mojito

Yes! There are keto-friendly cocktails. It takes a little preparation; stevia is used instead of sugar, but you don't need a blender. Muddling the mint leaves releases the mint fragrance and provides the minty backdrop for this refreshing drink. This is an easy recipe that is festive and interactive (muddling) for a fun part beverage.

Preparation Time: 15 minutes

Cooking Time: 30 minutes

Serves: 6

Ingredients

4 fresh mint leaves

2 T fresh lime Juice

2 t stevia

Ice

1.5 oz shot of white rum

splash club soda or plain seltzer

fresh mint as garnish

Directions:

Muddle the mint, lime juice, and stevia for 10 seconds in the glass in which the drink will be served.

Fill the glass with ice, either cubed or crushed.

Pour the shot of vodka over the ice.

Add club soda to fill the glass

Garnish with a mint leaf.

You may want to strain the drink after muddling to remove the broken mint leaves, so they don't get in the way of enjoying the drink. You can substitute vodka or gin for rum.

Nutrition:

Calories: 109

Carbohydrates: 2g

27. Chocolate Coconut Keto Smoothie Bowl

Preparation Time: 15 minutes

Cooking Time: 30 minutes

Serves: 6

Ingredients

1/3 cup vanilla protein powder

1 tbsp cocoa powder

1/4 cup walnuts

1/4 cup walnuts

1/2 cup almond milk

1 tbsp coconut oil

3 cup crushed ice

Sweetener

Directions:

Take a blender pour almond milk, protein powder, cocoa powder, sweetener and ice, blend the ingredients well. Now add coconut oil xanthan gum and blend until it increases in volume. Pour it into bowl adds fruits and nuts and serves.

Nutrition:

Calories per serving: 352

Carbohydrates: 2g

Protein: 42.5g

Fat: 42g

Sugar: 0.1g

Sodium: 152mg

Fiber: 0.7g

Conclusion

For some people, the ketogenic get-healthy plan is a phenomenal path for weight reduction. It is extraordinary and permits the person on the eating routine to devour an eating plan, which incorporates nourishments that you probably won't anticipate.

Along these lines, the ketogenic diet, or keto, is an eating plan that comprises of high fat and low carbs. Exactly what number of diet programs are there in which you can set up the free day with eggs and bacon, huge amounts of it, at that point take chicken wings for lunch and broccoli and steak for dinner.

That could sound too extraordinary to be in any way precise for some. Adequately on this specific eating routine, this is a phenomenal day of eating and you followed the rules totally with that supper program.

At whatever point you expend a little amount of sugars, the body is put into a condition of ketosis. This means the body can consume fat for vitality. Exactly how little of various carbs would you need to devour that can go into ketosis?Effectively, it differs for every person, though it is a safe option to remain under twenty-five total carbs. Most suggest that when you are in the "induction phase" that happens when you are really putting the body into ketosis, you must remain under ten total carbs.

Something to stress about when going on the ketogenic diet plan is a thing known as "keto flu. You will feel fatigued and you might have a headache. It will not last lengthy. If you are feeling by doing this, make certain you receive a lot of rest and water to overcome it.

Intermittent fasting has transformed into a most loved strategy to utilize your body's normal fat-copying ability to get in shape in a quick time. All things considered, numerous people wish to know, accomplishes discontinuous fasting work and exactly how precisely will it work?

At whatever point you go for a drawn out timeframe with no eating, the body changes the manner by which it produces proteins and hormones, which could be useful for weight reduction. These are the essential fasting benefits and the manner in which they achieve those advantages.

Hormones structure the establishment of metabolic stacks like the speed at which you consume off muscle versus fat. Development hormone is made by the body and energizes the breakdown of fat inside the body to give vitality.If you fast for quite a while, the body starts to improve the development hormone creation. Also, fasting attempts to diminish the amount of insulin contained in the circulatory system, ensuring that the body consumes fat as opposed to putting away it.

A momentary quick which keeps going 12-72 hours expands the metabolic procedure and adrenaline levels, making you support the quantity of calories consumed. Moreover, the individuals who quick furthermore acknowledge higher vitality through improved adrenaline, pushing them to not look depleted in spite of the fact that they are not getting calories regularly. While you may feel as fasting must prompt diminished vitality, the whole body makes up for this particular, guaranteeing a more unhealthy consuming daily schedule.

Almost all people that eat each 3-5 hours chiefly consume sugar as opposed to fat. Fasting for a significant stretch moves the digestion to losing fat. By the decision of a 24-hour fasting day, the body has just spent glycogen traders in two or three hours and has now invested around eighteen of the energy consuming by additional fat stores inside the body.

For anyone who is continually profitable, be that as it may, battles with weight reduction, irregular fasting can make it conceivable to support weight reduction without being compelled to increase an exercise design or definitely modify an eating routine program. An additional advantage of intermittent fasting is the fact that it resets an individual's body. Getting one day or even so without consuming changes an individual's craving, causing them to not really feel as starved after a while.

When you wrestle with consistently desiring food, intermittent fasting can assist your body to adjust to periods of refusing to eat and enable you to not really feel hungry continuously. Many people notice they begin eating healthier plus more controlled diets whenever they fast intermittently 1 day a week.

Intermittent fasting differs but is frequently recommended for approximately 1 day each week. During this working day, a person could have a nutrient-filled smoothie or any other low-calorie drink. As the entire body changes to an intermittent fasting program, this generally is not essential.

Intermittent fasting helps you to lessen body fat stores effortlessly in the entire body, by changing over the metabolism for breaking down body fat rather than muscle or sugar.

It has been used by many people effectively and it is a simple way to make an advantageous change. For anybody that struggles with stubborn fat and it is tired of regular dieting, intermittent fasting provides an effective and easy choice for weight loss and a healthier way of life.

If these two dieting patterns sound like the diet types, you will be interested in, then WHAT ARE YOU WAITING FOR?

Made in the USA
Monee, IL
27 May 2021